THE VEGETARIAN DIET

FOR WOMEN

Cookbook

The Best **100 recipes** to stay **TONE** and **HEALTHY**!
Reboot your Metabolism before Summer with the Tastiest
and Lightest **Plant-Based Meals**!

By

Jocelyn Grant

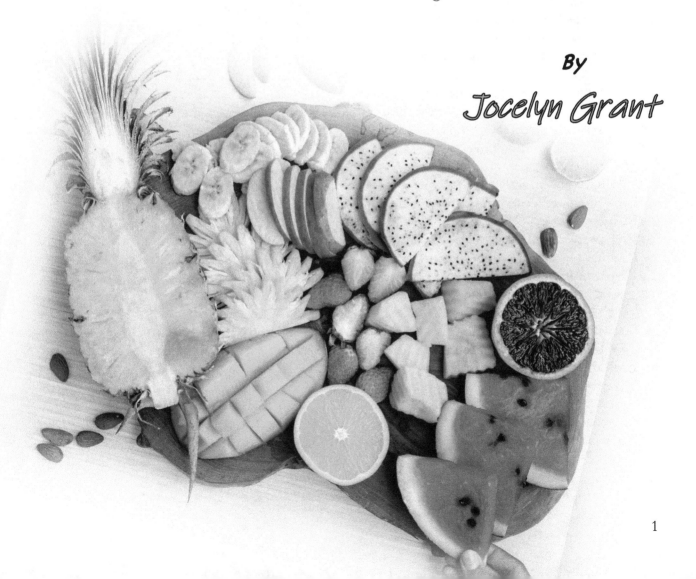

Table of Contents

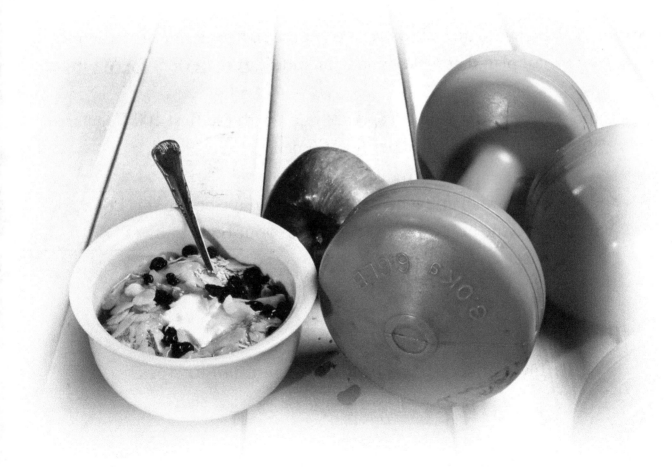

Introduction

In recent years, people have been thinking more and more about what they eat: they are concerned about eating healthy foods to provide the right nutrients to the body, but they are also interested in eating meals that are no full of preservatives or additives. People are increasingly concerned with eating less processed and more sustainable foods and this trend has turned many people into vegetarians or even vegans.

And a plant-based diet is really the best solution!

Because the Vegetarian diet allows you to get the right amount of nutrients and follow a meal plan that makes you light and fit, **it is perfect for Women**!

This is the reason why I created a specific book with the Best 100 Vegetarian Recipes for Women!

BONUS: Whit more than the best **100** Vegetarian recipes, in this book you will find also the best exercises to **TONE** your body to the **TOP**!

Ready to discover the best 100 Vegetarian Recipes?

LET'S GO!

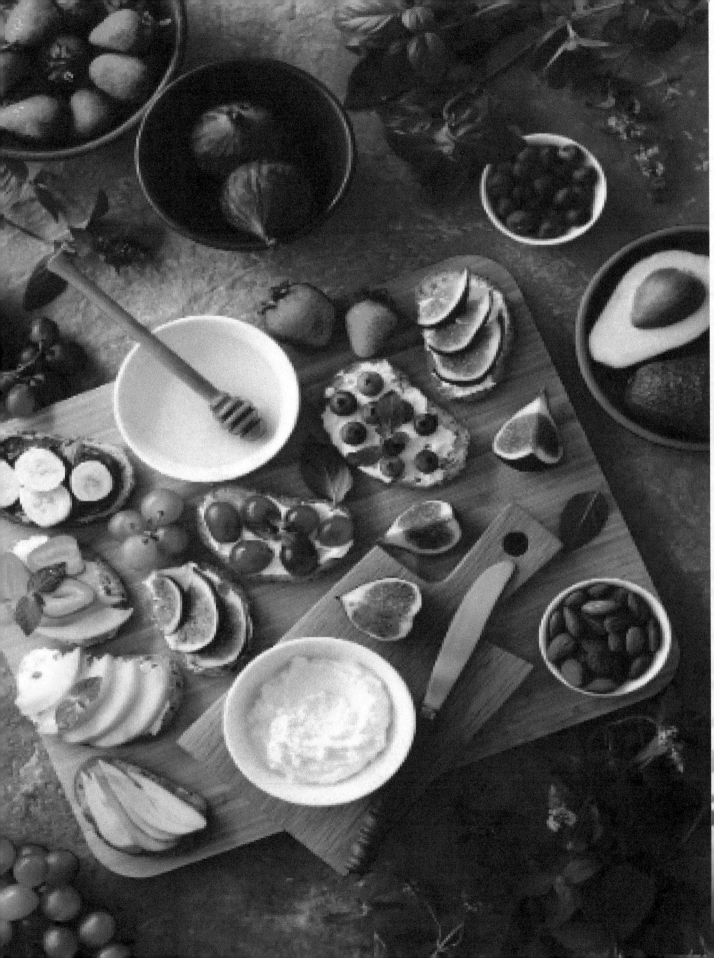

Chapter 1. BREAKFAST AND SNACKS

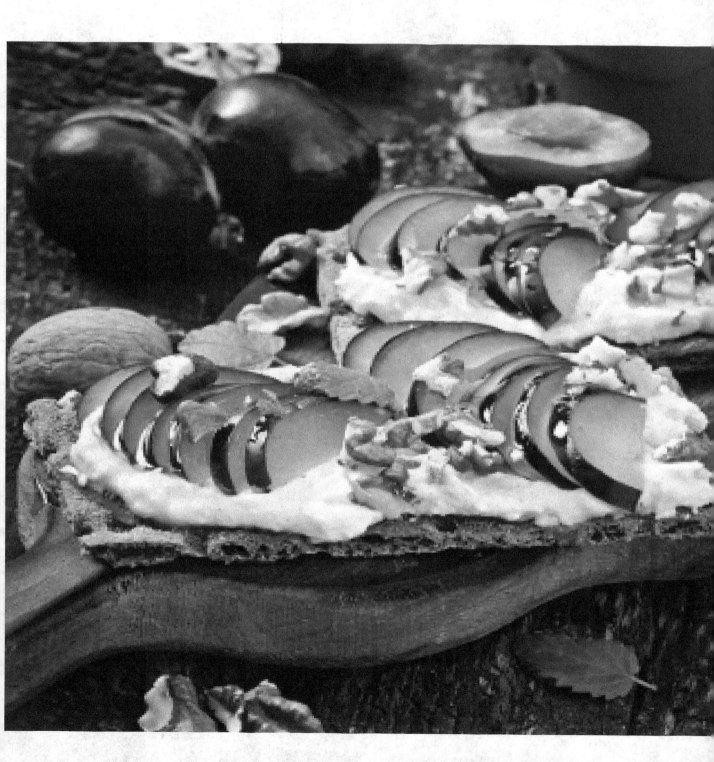

1) GREEK MUFFINS WITH TOFU ENGLISH RECIPE

Preparation Time: 15 minutes		Servings: 4

Ingredients:

- ✓ 2 tbsp olive oil
- ✓ 16 ounces extra-firm tofu
- ✓ 1 tbsp nutritional yeast
- ✓ 1/4 tsp turmeric powder
- ✓ 2 handfuls fresh kale, chopped
- ✓ Kosher salt and ground black pepper, to taste
- ✓ 4 English muffins, cut in half
- ✓ 4 tbsp ketchup
- ✓ 4 slices vegan cheese

Directions:

- ❖ Heat the olive oil in a frying skillet over medium heat. When it's hot, add the tofu and sauté for 8 minutes, stirring occasionally to promote even cooking.
- ❖ Add in the nutritional yeast, turmeric and kale and continue sautéing an additional 2 minutes or until the kale wilts. Season with salt and pepper to taste.
- ❖ Meanwhile, toast the English muffins until crisp.
- ❖ To assemble the sandwiches, spread the bottom halves of the English muffins with ketchup; top them with the tofu mixture and vegan cheese; place the bun topper on, close the sandwiches and serve warm.
- ❖ Enjoy

2) SPECIAL CINNAMON SEMOLINO PORRIDGE

Preparation Time: 20 minutes		Servings: 3

Ingredients:

- ✓ 3 cups almond milk
- ✓ 3 tbsp maple syrup
- ✓ 3 tsp coconut oil
- ✓ 1/4 tsp kosher salt
- ✓ 1/2 tsp ground cinnamon
- ✓ 1 ¼ cups semolina

Directions:

- ❖ In a saucepan, heat the almond milk, maple syrup, coconut oil, salt and cinnamon over a moderate flame.
- ❖ Once hot, gradually stir in the semolina flour. Turn the heat to a simmer and continue cooking until the porridge reaches your preferred consistency.
- ❖ Garnish with your favorite toppings and serve warm. Enjoy

3) EASY APPLESAUCE DECADENT FRENCH TOAST

Preparation Time: 15 minutes		Servings: 1

Ingredients:

- ✓ 1/4 cup oat milk, sweetened
- ✓ 2 tbsp applesauce, sweetened
- ✓ 1/2 tsp vanilla paste
- ✓ A pinch of salt
- ✓ A pinch of grated nutmeg
- ✓ 1/4 tsp ground cloves
- ✓ 1/4 tsp ground cinnamon
- ✓ 2 slices rustic day-old bread slices
- ✓ 1 tbsp coconut oil
- ✓ 1 tbsp maple syrup

Directions:

- ❖ In a mixing bowl, thoroughly combine the oat milk, applesauce, vanilla, salt, nutmeg, cloves and cinnamon.
- ❖ Dip each slice of bread into the custard mixture until well coated on all sides.
- ❖ Preheat the coconut oil in a frying pan over medium-high heat. Cook for about 3 minutes on each side, until golden brown.
- ❖ Drizzle the French toast with maple syrup and serve immediately. Enjoy

4) TASTY NUTTY BREAKFAST BREAD PUDDING

Preparation Time: 2 hours 10 minutes		Servings: 6

Ingredients:

- ✓ 1 ½ cups almond milk
- ✓ 1/2 cup maple syrup
- ✓ 2 tbsp almond butter
- ✓ 1/2 tsp vanilla extract
- ✓ 1/2 tsp almond extract
- ✓ 1/2 tsp ground cinnamon
- ✓ 1/2 tsp ground cloves
- ✓ 1/3 tsp kosher salt
- ✓ 1/2 cup almonds, roughly chopped
- ✓ 4 cups day-old white bread, cubed

Directions:

- ❖ In a mixing bowl, combine the almond milk, maple syrup, almond butter, vanilla extract, almond extract and spices.
- ❖ Add the bread cubes to the custard mixture and stir to combine well. Fold in the almonds and allow it to rest for about 1 hour.
- ❖ Then, spoon the mixture into a lightly oiled casserole dish.
- ❖ Bake in the preheated oven at 350 degrees F for about 1 hour or until the top is golden brown.
- ❖ Place the bread pudding on a wire rack for 10 minutes before slicing and serving. Enjoy

5) FRITTATA WITH MUSHROOMS AND PEPPERS

Preparation Time: 30 minutes		Servings: 4

Ingredients:

- ✓ 4 tbsp olive oil
- ✓ 1 red onion, minced
- ✓ 1 red bell pepper, sliced
- ✓ 1 tsp garlic, finely chopped
- ✓ 1 pound button mushrooms, sliced
- ✓ Sea salt and ground black pepper, to taste
- ✓ 1/2 tsp dried oregano
- ✓ 1/2 tsp dried dill
- ✓ 16 ounces tofu, drained and crumbled
- ✓ 2 tbsp nutritional yeast
- ✓ 1/2 tsp turmeric powder
- ✓ 4 tbsp corn flour
- ✓ 1/3 cup oat milk, unsweetened

Directions:

- ❖ Preheat 2 tbsp of the olive oil in a nonstick skillet over medium-high heat. Then, cook the onion and pepper for about 4 minutes until tender and fragrant.
- ❖ Add in the garlic and mushrooms and continue to sauté an additional 2 to 3 minutes or until aromatic. Season with salt, black pepper, oregano and dill. Reserve.
- ❖ In your blender or food processor, mix the tofu, nutritional yeast, turmeric powder, corn flour and milk. Process until you have a smooth and uniform paste.
- ❖ In the same skillet, heat 1 tbsp of the olive oil until sizzling. Pour in 1/2 of the tofu mixture and spread it with a spatula.
- ❖ Cook for about 6 minutes or until set; flip and cook it for another 3 minutes. Slide the omelet onto a serving plate.
- ❖ Spoon 1/2 of the mushroom filling over half of the omelet. Fold the unfilled half of omelet over the filling.
- ❖ Repeat with another omelet. Cut them into halves and serve warm. Enjoy

6) FROZEN HEMP AND BLACKBERRY SMOOTHIE BOWL

Preparation Time: 10 minutes		Servings: 2

Ingredients:

- ✓ 2 tbsp hemp seeds
- ✓ 1/2 cup coconut milk
- ✓ 1 cup coconut yogurt
- ✓ 1 cup blackberries, frozen
- ✓ 2 small-sized bananas, frozen
- ✓ 4 tbsp granola

Directions:

- ❖ In your blender, mix all ingredients, trying to keep the liquids at the bottom of the blender to help it break up the fruits.
- ❖ Divide your smoothie between serving bowls.
- ❖ Garnish each bowl with granola and some extra frozen berries, if desired. Serve immediately

7) DARK CHOCOLATE AND WALNUT STEEL-CUT OATS

Preparation Time: 30 minutes		Servings: 3

Ingredients:

- ✓ 2 cups oat milk
- ✓ 1/3 cup steel-cut oats
- ✓ 1 tbsp coconut oil
- ✓ 1/4 cup coconut sugar
- ✓ A pinch of grated nutmeg
- ✓ A pinch of flaky sea salt
- ✓ 1/4 tsp cinnamon powder
- ✓ 1/4 tsp vanilla extract
- ✓ 4 tbsp cocoa powder
- ✓ 1/3 cup English walnut halves
- ✓ 4 tbsp chocolate chips

Directions:

- ❖ Bring the oat milk and oats to a boil over a moderately high heat. Then, turn the heat to low and add in the coconut oil, sugar and spices; let it simmer for about 25 minutes, stirring periodically.
- ❖ Add in the cocoa powder and continue simmering an additional 3 minutes.
- ❖ Spoon the oatmeal into serving bowls. Top each bowl with the walnut halves and chocolate chips.
- ❖ Enjoy

8) EASY BUCKWHEAT PORRIDGE WITH APPLES-ALMONDS

Preparation Time: 20 minutes		Servings: 3

Ingredients:

- ✓ 1 cup buckwheat groats, toasted
- ✓ 3/4 cup water
- ✓ 1 cup rice milk
- ✓ 1/4 tsp sea salt
- ✓ 3 tbsp agave syrup
- ✓ 1 cup apples, cored and diced
- ✓ 3 tbsp almonds, slivered
- ✓ 2 tbsp coconut flakes
- ✓ 2 tbsp hemp seeds

Directions:

- ❖ In a saucepan, bring the buckwheat groats, water, milk and salt to a boil. Immediately turn the heat to a simmer; let it simmer for about 13 minutes until it has softened.
- ❖ Stir in the agave syrup. Divide the porridge between three serving bowls.
- ❖ Garnish each serving with the apples, almonds, coconut and hemp seeds. Enjoy

9) TRADITIONAL SPANISH TORTILLA

Preparation Time: 35 minutes | | **Servings:** 2

Ingredients:

- ✓ 3 tbsp olive oil
- ✓ 2 medium potatoes, peeled and diced
- ✓ 1/2 white onion, chopped
- ✓ 8 tbsp gram flour
- ✓ 8 tbsp water
- ✓ Sea salt and ground black pepper, to season
- ✓ 1/2 tsp Spanish paprika

Directions:

- ❖ Heat 2 tbsp of the olive oil in a frying pan over a moderate flame. Now, cook the potatoes and onion; cook for about 20 minutes or until tender; reserve.
- ❖ In a mixing bowl, thoroughly combine the flour, water, salt, black pepper and paprika. Add in the potato/onion mixture.
- ❖ Heat the remaining 1 tbsp of the olive oil in the same frying pan. Pour 1/2 of the batter into the frying pan. Cook your tortilla for about 11 minutes, turning it once or twice to promote even cooking.
- ❖ Repeat with the remaining batter and serve warm

10) SPECIAL CHOCOLATE AND MANGO QUINOA BOWL

Preparation Time: 35 minutes | | **Servings:** 2

Ingredients:

- ✓ 1 cup quinoa
- ✓ 1 tsp ground cinnamon
- ✓ 1 cup non-dairy milk
- ✓ 1 large mango, chopped
- ✓ 3 tbsp unsweetened cocoa powder
- ✓ 2 tbsp almond butter
- ✓ 1 tbsp hemp seeds
- ✓ 1 tbsp walnuts
- ✓ ¼ cup raspberries

Directions:

- ❖ In a pot, combine the quinoa, cinnamon, milk, and 1 cup of water over medium heat. Bring to a boil, low heat, and simmer covered for 25-30 minutes. In a bowl, mash the mango and mix cocoa powder, almond butter, and hemp seeds. In a serving bowl, place cooked quinoa and mango mixture.
- ❖ Top with walnuts and raspberries. Serve immediately

11) EASY ORANGE AND CARROT MUFFINS WITH CHERRIES

Preparation Time: 45 minutes | | **Servings:** 6

Ingredients:

- ✓ 1 tsp vegetable oil
- ✓ 2 tbsp almond butter
- ✓ ¼ cup non-dairy milk
- ✓ 1 orange, peeled
- ✓ 1 carrot, coarsely chopped
- ✓ 2 tbsp chopped dried cherries
- ✓ 3 tbsp molasses
- ✓ 2 tbsp ground flaxseed
- ✓ 1 tsp apple cider vinegar
- ✓ 1 tsp pure vanilla extract
- ✓ ½ tsp ground cinnamon
- ✓ ½ tsp ground ginger
- ✓ ¼ tsp ground nutmeg
- ✓ ¼ tsp allspice
- ✓ ¾ cup whole-wheat flour
- ✓ 1 tsp baking powder
- ✓ ½ tsp baking soda
- ✓ ½ cup rolled oats
- ✓ 2 tbsp raisins
- ✓ 2 tbsp sunflower seeds

Directions:

- ❖ Preheat oven to 350 F. Grease 6 muffin cups with vegetable oil.
- ❖ In a food processor, add the almond butter, milk, orange, carrot, cherries, molasses, flaxseed, vinegar, vanilla, cinnamon, ginger, nutmeg, and allspice and blend until smooth.
- ❖ In a bowl, combine the flour, baking powder, and baking soda. Fold in the wet mixture and gently stir to combine. Mix in the oats, raisins, and sunflower seeds. Divide the batter between muffin cups. Put in a baking tray and bake for 30 minutes

12) SIMPLE QUINOA LEMONY MUFFINS

Preparation Time: 25 minutes		Servings: 5

Ingredients:

- ✓ 2 tbsp coconut oil melted, plus more for coating the muffin tin
- ✓ ¼ cup ground flaxseed
- ✓ 2 cups unsweetened lemon curd
- ✓ ½ cup pure date sugar
- ✓ 1 tsp apple cider vinegar
- ✓ 2 ½ cups whole-wheat flour
- ✓ 1 ½ cups cooked quinoa
- ✓ 2 tsp baking soda
- ✓ A pinch of salt
- ✓ ½ cup raisins

Directions:

- ❖ Preheat oven to 400 F.
- ❖ In a bowl, combine the flaxseed and ½ cup water. Stir in the lemon curd, sugar, coconut oil, and vinegar. Add in flour, quinoa, baking soda, and salt. Put in the raisins, be careful not too fluffy.
- ❖ Divide the batter between greased with coconut oil cups of the tin and bake for 20 minutes until golden and set. Allow cooling slightly before removing it from the tin. Serve

13) RICH OATMEAL ALMOND PORRIDGE

Preparation Time: 25 minutes		Servings: 4

Ingredients:

- ✓ 2 ½ cups vegetable broth
- ✓ 2 ½ cups almond milk
- ✓ ½ cup steel-cut oats
- ✓ 1 tbsp pearl barley
- ✓ ½ cup slivered almonds
- ✓ ¼ cup nutritional yeast
- ✓ 2 cups old-fashioned rolled oats

Directions:

- ❖ • Pour the broth and almond milk in a pot over medium heat and bring to a boil. Stir in oats, pearl barley, almond slivers, and nutritional yeast. Reduce the heat and simmer for 20 minutes. Add in the rolled oats, cook for an additional 5 minutes, until creamy. Allow cooling before serving

14) RICH BREAKFAST PECAN AND PEAR FARRO

Preparation Time: 20 minutes		Servings: 4

Ingredients:

- ✓ 2 cups water
- ✓ ½ tsp salt
- ✓ 1 cup farro
- ✓ 1 tbsp plant butter
- ✓ 2 pears, peeled, cored, and chopped
- ✓ ¼ cup chopped pecans

Directions:

- ❖ Bring water to a boil in a pot over high heat. Stir in salt and farro. Lower the heat, cover, and simmer for 15 minutes until the farro is tender and the liquid has absorbed. Turn the heat off and add in the butter, pears, and pecans. Cover and rest for 12-15 minutes.
- ❖ Serve immediately

15) SIMPLE BLACKBERRY WAFFLES

Preparation Time: 15 minutes | | **Servings: 4**

Ingredients:

- ✓ 1 ½ cups whole-heat flour
- ✓ ½ cup old-fashioned oats
- ✓ ¼ cup date sugar
- ✓ 3 tsp baking powder
- ✓ ½ tsp salt
- ✓ 1 tsp ground cinnamon
- ✓ 2 cups soy milk
- ✓ 1 tbsp fresh lemon juice
- ✓ 1 tsp lemon zest
- ✓ ¼ cup plant butter, melted
- ✓ ½ cup fresh blackberries

Directions:

- ❖ Preheat the waffle iron.
- ❖ In a bowl, mix flour, oats, sugar, baking powder, salt, and cinnamon. Set aside. In another bowl, combine milk, lemon juice, lemon zest, and butter. Pour into the wet ingredients and whisk to combine. Add the batter to the hot greased waffle iron, using approximately a ladleful for each waffle. Cook for 3-5 minutes, until golden brown. Repeat the process until no batter is left.
- ❖ Serve topped with blackberries

16) AUTHENTIC WALNUT WAFFLES WITH MAPLE SYRUP

Preparation Time: 15 minutes | | **Servings: 4**

Ingredients:

- ✓ 1 ¾ cups whole-wheat flour
- ✓ ⅓ cup coarsely ground walnuts
- ✓ 1 tbsp baking powder
- ✓ 1 ½p cups soy milk
- ✓ 3 tbsp pure maple syrup
- ✓ 3 tbsp plant butter, melted

Directions:

- ❖ Preheat the waffle iron and grease with oil. Combine the flour, walnuts, baking powder, and salt in a bowl. Set aside. In another bowl, mix the milk and butter. Pour into the walnut mixture and whisk until well combined. Spoon a ladleful of the batter onto the waffle iron.
- ❖ Cook for 3-5 minutes, until golden brown. Repeat the process until no batter is left. Top with maple syrup to serve

18) SIMPLE ORANGE AND BRAN CUPS WITH DATES

Preparation Time: 30 minutes		**Servings: 12**

Ingredients:

- ✓ 1 tsp vegetable oil
- ✓ 3 cups bran flakes cereal
- ✓ 1 ½ cups whole-wheat flour
- ✓ ½ cup dates, chopped
- ✓ 3 tsp baking powder
- ✓ ½ tsp ground cinnamon
- ✓ ½ tsp salt
- ✓ ⅓ cup brown sugar
- ✓ ¾ cup fresh orange juice

Directions:

- ❖ Preheat oven to 400 F. Grease a 12-cup muffin tin with oil.
- ❖ Mix the bran flakes, flour, dates, baking powder, cinnamon, and salt in a bowl. In another bowl, combine the sugar and orange juice until blended. Pour into the dry mixture and whisk. Divide the mixture between the cups of the muffin tin. Bake for 20 minutes or until golden brown and set. Cool for a few minutes before removing from the tin and serve

19) EXOTIC MACADAMIA NUTS AND APPLE-DATE COUSCOUS

Preparation Time: 20 minutes		**Servings: 4**

Ingredients:

- ✓ 3 cups apple juice
- ✓ 1 ½ cups couscous
- ✓ 1 tsp ground cinnamon
- ✓ ¼ tsp ground cloves
- ✓ ½ cup dried dates
- ✓ ½ cup chopped macadamia nuts

Directions:

- ❖ Pour the apple juice into a pot over medium heat and bring to a boil. Stir in couscous, cinnamon, and cloves. Turn the heat off and cover. Let sit for 5 minutes until the liquid is absorbed.
- ❖ Using a fork, fluff the couscous and add the dates and macadamia nuts, stir to combine. Serve warm

20) TASTY BLUEBERRY COCONUT MUFFINS

Preparation Time: 30 minutes		**Servings: 12**

Ingredients:

- ✓ 1 tbsp coconut oil melted
- ✓ 1 cup quick-cooking oats
- ✓ 1 cup boiling water
- ✓ ½ cup almond milk
- ✓ ¼ cup ground flaxseed
- ✓ 1 tsp almond extract
- ✓ 1 tsp apple cider vinegar
- ✓ 1 ½ cups whole-wheat flour
- ✓ ½ cup pure date sugar
- ✓ 2 tsp baking soda
- ✓ A pinch of salt
- ✓ 1 cup blueberries

Directions:

- ❖ Preheat oven to 400 F.
- ❖ In a bowl, stir in the oats with boiling water until they are softened. Pour in the coconut oil, milk, flaxseed, almond extract, and vinegar. Add in the flour, sugar, baking soda, and salt. Gently stir in blueberries.
- ❖ Divide the batter between a greased with coconut oil muffin tin. Bake for 20 minutes until lightly brown. Allow cooling for 10 minutes. Using a spatula, run the sides of the muffins to take out. Serve

21) SWISS-STYLE CHARD SCRAMBLED TOFU

Preparation Time: 35 minutes

Servings: 5

Ingredients:

- ✓ 1 (14-oz) package tofu, crumbled
- ✓ 2 tsp olive oil
- ✓ 1 onion, chopped
- ✓ 3 cloves minced garlic
- ✓ 1 celery stalk, chopped
- ✓ 2 large carrots, chopped
- ✓ 1 tsp chili powder
- ✓ ½ tsp ground cumin
- ✓ ½ tsp ground turmeric
- ✓ Salt and black pepper to taste
- ✓ 5 cups Swiss chard

Directions:

- ❖ Heat the oil in a skillet over medium heat. Add in the onion, garlic, celery, and carrots. Sauté for 5 minutes. Stir in tofu, chili powder, cumin, turmeric, salt, and pepper, cook for 7-8 minutes more.
- ❖ Mix in the Swiss chard and cook until wilted, about 3 minutes. Allow cooling and seal and serve

Chapter 2. LUNCH

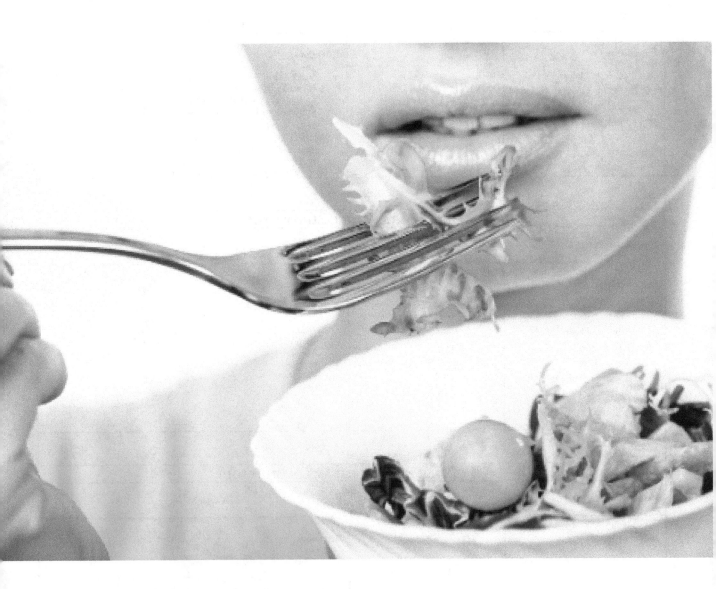

22) ITALIAN SPINACH AND KALE SOUP WITH FRIED COLLARDS

Preparation Time: 16 minutes | | **Servings:** 4

Ingredients:

- 4 tbsp plant butter
- 1 cup fresh spinach, chopped
- 1 cup fresh kale, chopped
- 1 large avocado
- 3 ½ cups coconut cream
- 4 cups vegetable broth
- 3 tbsp chopped fresh mint leaves
- Salt and black pepper to taste
- Juice from 1 lime
- 1 cup collard greens, chopped
- 2 garlic cloves, minced
- 1 pinch of green cardamom powder

Directions:

- Melt 2 tbsp of plant butter in a saucepan over medium heat and sauté spinach and kale for 5 minutes. Turn the heat off. Add the avocado, coconut cream, vegetable broth, salt, and pepper. Puree the ingredients with an immersion blender until smooth. Pour in the lime juice and set aside.
- Melt the remaining plant butter in a pan and add the collard greens, garlic, and cardamom; sauté until the garlic is fragrant and has achieved a golden brown color, about 4 minutes. Fetch the soup into serving bowls and garnish with fried collards and mint. Serve warm

23) HUNGARIAN GOULASH TOFU SOUP

Preparation Time: 25 minutes | | **Servings:** 4

Ingredients:

- 1 ½ cups extra-firm tofu, crumbled
- 3 tbsp plant butter
- 1 white onion
- 2 garlic cloves
- 8 oz chopped butternut squash
- 1 red bell pepper
- 1 tbsp paprika powder
- ¼ tsp red chili flakes
- 1 tbsp dried basil
- ½ tbsp crushed cardamom seeds
- Salt and black pepper to taste
- 1 ½ cups crushed tomatoes
- 4 cups vegetable broth
- 1 ½ tsp red wine vinegar
- Chopped cilantro to serve

Directions:

- Melt plant butter in a pot over medium heat and sauté onion and garlic for 3 minutes. Stir in tofu and cook for 3 minutes; add the butternut squash, bell pepper, paprika, red chili flakes, basil, cardamom seeds, salt, and pepper. Cook for 2 minutes. Pour in tomatoes and vegetable broth. Bring to a boil, reduce the heat and simmer for 10 minutes. Mix in red wine vinegar. Garnish with cilantro and serve

24) WINTER PUMPKIN CREAM COCONUT SOUP

Preparation Time: 55 minutes | | **Servings:** 4

Ingredients:

- 2 small red onions, cut into wedges
- 2 garlic cloves, skinned
- 10 oz pumpkin, cubed
- 10 oz butternut squash
- 2 tbsp olive oil
- 4 tbsp plant butter
- Juice of 1 lime
- ¾ cup tofu mayonnaise
- Toasted pumpkin seeds for garnish

Directions:

- Preheat oven to 400 F.
- Place onions, garlic, and pumpkin in a baking sheet and drizzle with olive oil. Season with salt and pepper. Roast for 30 minutes or until the vegetables are golden brown and fragrant. Remove the vegetables from the oven and transfer to a pot. Add 2 cups of water, bring the ingredients to boil over medium heat for 15 minutes. Turn the heat off. Add in plant butter and puree until smooth. Stir in lime juice and tofu mayonnaise. Spoon into serving bowls and garnish with pumpkin seeds to serve

25) ALL SEASONS CELERY AND POTATO SOUP

Preparation Time: 55 minutes | | **Servings:** 6

Ingredients:

- ✓ 2 tbsp olive oil
- ✓ 1 onion, chopped
- ✓ 1 carrot, chopped
- ✓ 1 celery stalk, chopped
- ✓ 2 garlic cloves, minced
- ✓ 1 golden beet, peeled and diced
- ✓ 1 yellow bell pepper, chopped
- ✓ 1 Yukon Gold potato, diced
- ✓ 6 cups vegetable broth
- ✓ 1 tsp dried thyme
- ✓ Salt and black pepper to taste
- ✓ 1 tbsp lemon juice

Directions:

❖ Heat the oil in a pot over medium heat. Place the onion, carrot, celery, and garlic. Cook for 5 minutes or until softened. Stir in beet, bell pepper, and potato, cook uncovered for 1 minute. Pour in the broth and thyme. Season with salt and pepper. Cook for 45 minutes until the vegetables are tender. Serve sprinkled with lemon juice

26) ITALIAN MUSHROOM SOUP OF MEDLEY

Preparation Time: 40 minutes | | **Servings:** 4

Ingredients:

- ✓ 4 oz unsalted plant butter
- ✓ 1 small onion, finely chopped
- ✓ 1 clove garlic, minced
- ✓ 5 oz button mushrooms, chopped
- ✓ 5 oz cremini mushrooms, chopped
- ✓ 5 oz shiitake mushrooms, chopped
- ✓ ½ lb celery root, chopped
- ✓ ½ tsp dried rosemary
- ✓ 1 vegetable stock cube, crushed
- ✓ 1 tbsp plain vinegar
- ✓ 1 cup coconut cream
- ✓ 4 – 6 leaves basil, chopped

Directions:

❖ Place a saucepan over medium-high heat, add the plant butter to melt, then sauté the onion, garlic, mushrooms, and celery root in the butter until golden brown and fragrant, about 6 minutes. Fetch out some mushrooms and reserve for garnishing. Add the rosemary, 3 cups of water, stock cube, and vinegar. Stir the mixture and bring it to a boil for 6 minutes. After, reduce the heat and simmer the soup for 15 minutes or until the celery is soft.

❖ Mix in the coconut cream and puree the ingredients using an immersion blender. Simmer for 2 minutes. Spoon the soup into serving bowls, garnish with the reserved mushrooms and basil. Serve

27) MEDITERRANEAN DILL CAULIFLOWER SOUP

Preparation Time: 26 minutes | | **Servings:** 4

Ingredients:

- ✓ 2 tbsp coconut oil
- ✓ ½ lb celery root, trimmed
- ✓ 1 garlic clove
- ✓ 1 medium white onion
- ✓ ¼ cup fresh dill, roughly chopped
- ✓ 1 tsp cumin powder
- ✓ ¼ tsp nutmeg powder
- ✓ 1 head cauliflower, cut into florets
- ✓ 3 ½ cups seasoned vegetable stock
- ✓ 5 oz plant butter
- ✓ Juice from 1 lemon
- ✓ ¼ cup coconut whipping cream

Directions:

❖ Set a pot over medium heat, add the coconut oil and allow heating until no longer shimmering.

❖ Add the celery root, garlic clove, and onion; sauté the vegetables until fragrant and soft, about 5 minutes. Stir in the dill, cumin, and nutmeg, and fry further for 1 minute. Mix in the cauliflower florets and vegetable stock. Bring the soup to a boil for 12 to 15 minutes or until the cauliflower is soft. Turn the heat off. Add the plant butter and lemon juice. Puree the ingredients with an immersion blender until smooth. Mix in coconut whipping cream and season the soup with salt and black pepper. Serve warm

28) SPECIAL FENNEL BROCCOLI SOUP

Preparation Time: 25 minutes | | **Servings:** 4

Ingredients:

- ✓ 1 fennel bulb, chopped
- ✓ 10 oz broccoli, cut into florets
- ✓ 3 cups vegetable stock
- ✓ Salt and black pepper to taste
- ✓ 1 garlic clove
- ✓ 1 cup cashew cream cheese
- ✓ 3 oz plant butter
- ✓ ½ cup chopped fresh oregano

Directions:

- ❖ Put the fennel and broccoli into a pot, and cover with the vegetable stock. Bring the ingredients to a boil over medium heat until the vegetables are soft, about 10 minutes. Season the liquid with salt and black pepper, and drop in the garlic. Simmer the soup for 5 to 7 minutes and turn the heat off.
- ❖ Pour the cream cheese, plant butter, and oregano into the soup; puree the ingredients with an immersion blender until completely smooth. Adjust the taste with salt and black pepper. Spoon the soup into serving bowls and serve

29) EASY BEAN SOUP ASIAN-STYLE

Preparation Time: 55 minutes | | **Servings:** 4

Ingredients:

- ✓ 1 cup canned cannellini beans
- ✓ 2 tsp curry powder
- ✓ 2 tsp olive oil
- ✓ 1 red onion, diced
- ✓ 1 tbsp minced fresh ginger
- ✓ 2 cubed sweet potatoes
- ✓ 1 cup sliced zucchini
- ✓ Salt and black pepper to taste
- ✓ 4 cups vegetable stock
- ✓ 1 bunch spinach, chopped
- ✓ Toasted sesame seeds

Directions:

- ❖ Mix the beans with 1 tsp of curry powder until well combined. Warm the oil in a pot over medium heat. Place the onion and ginger and cook for 5 minutes until soft. Add in sweet potatoes and cook for 10 minutes. Put in zucchini and cook for 5 minutes. Season with the remaining curry, pepper, and salt.
- ❖ Pour in the stock and bring to a boil. Lower the heat and simmer for 25 minutes. Stir in beans and spinach. Cook until the spinach wilts and remove from the heat. Garnish with sesame seeds to serve

30) TORTILLA MEXICAN-STYLE SOUP

Preparation Time: 40 minutes | | **Servings:** 4

Ingredients:

- ✓ 1 (14.5-oz) can diced tomatoes
- ✓ 1 (4-oz) can green chiles, chopped
- ✓ 2 tbsp olive oil
- ✓ 1 cup canned sweet corn
- ✓ 1 red onion, chopped
- ✓ 2 garlic cloves, minced
- ✓ 2 jalapeño peppers, sliced
- ✓ 4 cups vegetable broth
- ✓ 8 oz seitan, cut into ¼-inch strips
- ✓ Salt and black pepper to taste
- ✓ ¼ cup chopped fresh cilantro
- ✓ 3 tbsp fresh lime juice
- ✓ 4 corn tortillas, cut into strips
- ✓ 1 ripe avocado, chopped

Directions:

- ❖ Preheat oven to 350 F. Heat the oil in a pot over medium heat. Place sweet corn, garlic, jalapeño, and onion and cook for 5 minutes. Stir in broth, seitan, tomatoes, canned chiles, salt, and pepper. Bring to a boil, then lower the heat and simmer for 20 minutes. Put in the cilantro and lime juice, stir. Adjust the seasoning.
- ❖ Meanwhile, arrange the tortilla strips on a baking sheet and bake for 8 minutes until crisp. Serve the soup into bowls and top with tortilla strips and avocado

31) HOT BEAN SPICY SOUP

Preparation Time: 40 minutes		Servings: 4

Ingredients:

- ✓ 2 tbsp olive oil
- ✓ 1 medium onion, chopped
- ✓ 2 large garlic cloves, minced
- ✓ 1 carrot, chopped
- ✓ 1 (15.5-oz) can cannellini beans, drained
- ✓ 5 cups vegetable broth
- ✓ ¼ tsp crushed red pepper
- ✓ Salt and black pepper to taste
- ✓ 3 cups chopped baby spinach

Directions:

❖ Heat oil in a pot over medium heat. Place in carrot, onion, and garlic and cook for 3 minutes. Put in beans, broth, red pepper, salt, and black pepper and stir. Bring to a boil, then lower the heat and simmer for 25 minutes. Stir in baby spinach and cook for 5 minutes until the spinach wilts. Serve warm

32) SPECIAL MUSHROOM RICE WINE SOUP

Preparation Time: 25 minutes		Servings: 4

Ingredients:

- ✓ 2 tbsp olive oil
- ✓ 4 green onions, chopped
- ✓ 1 carrot, chopped
- ✓ 8 oz shiitake mushrooms, sliced
- ✓ 3 tbsp rice wine
- ✓ 2 tbsp soy sauce
- ✓ 4 cups vegetable broth
- ✓ Salt and black pepper to taste
- ✓ 2 tbsp parsley, chopped

Directions:

❖ Heat the oil in a pot over medium heat. Place the green onions and carrot and cook for 5 minutes.

❖ Stir in mushrooms, rice wine, soy sauce, broth, salt, and pepper. Bring to a boil, then lower the heat and simmer for 15 minutes. Top with parsley and serve warm

33) TASTY BEAN TANGY TOMATO SOUP

Preparation Time: 30 minutes		Servings: 5

Ingredients:

- ✓ 2 tsp olive oil
- ✓ 1 onion, chopped
- ✓ 2 garlic cloves, minced
- ✓ 1 cup mushrooms, chopped
- ✓ Sea salt to taste
- ✓ 1 tbsp dried basil
- ✓ ½ tbsp dried oregano
- ✓ 1 (19-oz) can diced tomatoes
- ✓ 1 (14-oz) can kidney beans, drained
- ✓ 5 cups water
- ✓ 2 cups chopped mustard greens

Directions:

❖ Heat the oil in a pot over medium heat. Place in the onion, garlic, mushrooms, and salt and cook for 5 minutes. Stir in basil and oregano, tomatoes, and beans. Pour in water and stir. Simmer for 20 minutes and add in mustard greens; cook for 5 minutes until greens soften. Serve immediately

34) EASY SPINACH AND POTATO SOUP

Preparation Time: 55 minutes		Servings: 4

Ingredients:

- 2 tbsp olive oil
- 1 onion, chopped
- 2 garlic cloves, minced
- 4 cups vegetable broth
- 2 russet potatoes, cubed
- ½ tsp dried oregano
- ¼ tsp crushed red pepper
- 1 bay leaf
- Salt to taste
- 4 cups chopped spinach
- 1 cup green lentils, rinsed

Directions:

❖ Warm the oil in a pot over medium heat. Place the onion and garlic and cook covered for 5 minutes. Stir in broth, potatoes, oregano, red pepper, bay leaf, lentils, and salt. Bring to a boil, then lower the heat and simmer uncovered for 30 minutes. Add in spinach and cook for another 5 minutes. Discard the bay leaf and serve immediately

35) MEXICAN BEAN TURMERIC SOUP

Preparation Time: 50 minutes		Servings: 6

Ingredients:

- 3 tbsp olive oil
- 1 onion, chopped
- 2 carrots, chopped
- 1 sweet potato, chopped
- 1 yellow bell pepper, chopped
- 2 garlic cloves, minced
- 4 tomatoes, chopped
- 6 cups vegetable broth
- 1 bay leaf
- Salt to taste
- 1 tsp ground cayenne pepper
- 1 (15.5-oz) can white beans, drained
- ⅓ cup whole-wheat pasta
- ¼ tsp turmeric

Directions:

❖ Heat the oil in a pot over medium heat. Place onion, carrots, sweet potato, bell pepper, and garlic. Cook for 5 minutes. Add in tomatoes, broth, bay leaf, salt, and cayenne pepper. Stir and bring to a boil. Lower the heat and simmer for 10 minutes. Put in white beans and simmer for 15 more minutes.

❖ Cook the pasta in a pot with boiling salted water and turmeric for 8-10 minutes, until pasta is al dente. Strain and transfer to the soup. Discard the bay leaf. Spoon into a bowl and serve

36) TROPICAL COCONUT ARUGULA SOUP

Preparation Time: 30 minutes		Servings: 4

Ingredients:

- 1 tsp coconut oil
- 1 onion, diced
- 2 cups green beans
- 4 cups water
- 1 cup arugula, chopped
- 1 tbsp fresh mint, chopped
- Sea salt and black pepper to taste
- ¾ cup coconut milk

Directions:

❖ Place a pot over medium heat and heat the coconut oil. Add in the onion and sauté for 5 minutes. Pour in green beans and water. Bring to a boil, lower the heat and stir in arugula, mint, salt, and pepper. Simmer for 10 minutes. Stir in coconut milk. Transfer to a food processor and blitz the soup until smooth. Serve

37) AUTHENTIC LENTIL SOUP WITH SWISS CHARD

Preparation Time: 25 minutes

Servings: 5

Ingredients:

- ✓ 2 tbsp olive oil
- ✓ 1 white onion, chopped
- ✓ 1 tsp garlic, minced
- ✓ 2 large carrots, chopped
- ✓ 1 parsnip, chopped
- ✓ 2 stalks celery, chopped
- ✓ 2 bay leaves
- ✓ 1/2 tsp dried thyme
- ✓ 1/4 tsp ground cumin
- ✓ 5 cups roasted vegetable broth
- ✓ 1 ¼ cups brown lentils, soaked overnight and rinsed
- ✓ 2 cups Swiss chard, torn into pieces

Directions:

- ❖ In a heavy-bottomed pot, heat the olive oil over a moderate heat. Now, sauté the vegetables along with the spices for about 3 minutes until they are just tender.
- ❖ Add in the vegetable broth and lentils, bringing it to a boil. Immediately turn the heat to a simmer and add in the bay leaves. Let it cook for about 15 minutes or until lentils are tender.
- ❖ Add in the Swiss chard, cover and let it simmer for 5 minutes more or until the chard wilts.
- ❖ Serve in individual bowls and enjoy

38) AUTUMN SPICY FARRO SOUP

Preparation Time: 30 minutes

Servings: 4

Ingredients:

- ✓ 2 tbsp olive oil
- ✓ 1 medium-sized leek, chopped
- ✓ 1 medium-sized turnip, sliced
- ✓ 2 Italian peppers, seeded and chopped
- ✓ 1 jalapeno pepper, minced
- ✓ 2 potatoes, peeled and diced
- ✓ 4 cups vegetable broth
- ✓ 1 cup farro, rinsed
- ✓ 1/2 tsp granulated garlic
- ✓ 1/2 tsp turmeric powder
- ✓ 1 bay laurel
- ✓ 2 cups spinach, turn into pieces

Directions:

- ❖ In a heavy-bottomed pot, heat the olive oil over a moderate heat. Now, sauté the leek, turnip, peppers and potatoes for about 5 minutes until they are crisp-tender.
- ❖ Add in the vegetable broth, farro, granulated garlic, turmeric and bay laurel; bring it to a boil.
- ❖ Immediately turn the heat to a simmer. Let it cook for about 25 minutes or until farro and potatoes have softened.
- ❖ Add in the spinach and remove the pot from the heat; let the spinach sit in the residual heat until it wilts. Enjoy

39) ALL COLORED CHICKPEA SALAD

Preparation Time: 30 minutes

Servings: 4

Ingredients:

- ✓ 16 ounces canned chickpeas, drained
- ✓ 1 medium avocado, sliced
- ✓ 1 bell pepper, seeded and sliced
- ✓ 1 large tomato, sliced
- ✓ 2 cucumber, diced
- ✓ 1 red onion, sliced
- ✓ 1/2 tsp garlic, minced
- ✓ 1/4 cup fresh parsley, chopped
- ✓ 1/4 cup olive oil
- ✓ 2 tbsp apple cider vinegar
- ✓ 1/2 lime, freshly squeezed
- ✓ Sea salt and ground black pepper, to taste

Directions:

- ❖ Toss all the ingredients in a salad bowl.
- ❖ Place the salad in your refrigerator for about 1 hour before serving.
- ❖ Enjoy

40) MEDITERRANEAN-STYLE LENTIL SALAD

Preparation Time: 20 minutes + chilling time		Servings: 5

Ingredients:

- ✓ 1 ½ cups red lentil, rinsed
- ✓ 1 tsp deli mustard
- ✓ 1/2 lemon, freshly squeezed
- ✓ 2 tbsp tamari sauce
- ✓ 2 scallion stalks, chopped
- ✓ 1/4 cup extra-virgin olive oil
- ✓ 2 garlic cloves, minced
- ✓ 1 cup butterhead lettuce, torn into pieces
- ✓ 2 tbsp fresh parsley, chopped
- ✓ 2 tbsp fresh cilantro, chopped
- ✓ 1 tsp fresh basil
- ✓ 1 tsp fresh oregano
- ✓ 1 ½ cups cherry tomatoes, halved
- ✓ 3 ounces Kalamata olives, pitted and halved

Directions:

- ❖ In a large-sized saucepan, bring 4 ½ cups of the water and the red lentils to a boil.
- ❖ Immediately turn the heat to a simmer and continue to cook your lentils for about 15 minutes or until tender. Drain and let it cool completely.
- ❖ Transfer the lentils to a salad bowl; toss the lentils with the remaining ingredients until well combined.
- ❖ Serve chilled or at room temperature. Enjoy

41) DELICIOUS ROASTED AVOCADO AND ASPARAGUS SALAD

Preparation Time: 20 minutes + chilling time		Servings: 4

Ingredients:

- ✓ 1 pound asparagus, trimmed, cut into bite-sized pieces
- ✓ 1 white onion, chopped
- ✓ 2 garlic cloves, minced
- ✓ 1 Roma tomato, sliced
- ✓ 1/4 cup olive oil
- ✓ 1/4 cup balsamic vinegar
- ✓ 1 tbsp stone-ground mustard
- ✓ 2 tbsp fresh parsley, chopped
- ✓ 1 tbsp fresh cilantro, chopped
- ✓ 1 tbsp fresh basil, chopped
- ✓ Sea salt and ground black pepper, to taste
- ✓ 1 small avocado, pitted and diced
- ✓ 1/2 cup pine nuts, roughly chopped

Directions:

- ❖ Begin by preheating your oven to 420 degrees F.
- ❖ Toss the asparagus with 1 tbsp of the olive oil and arrange them on a parchment-lined roasting pan.
- ❖ Bake for about 15 minutes, rotating the pan once or twice to promote even cooking. Let it cool completely and place in your salad bowl.
- ❖ Toss the asparagus with the vegetables, olive oil, vinegar, mustard and herbs. Salt and pepper to taste.
- ❖ Toss to combine and top with avocado and pine nuts. Enjoy

42) SPECIAL GREEN BEAN CREAM SALAD WITH PINE NUTS

Preparation Time: 10 minutes + chilling time		Servings: 5

Ingredients:

- ✓ 1 ½ pounds green beans, trimmed
- ✓ 2 medium tomatoes, diced
- ✓ 2 bell peppers, seeded and diced
- ✓ 4 tbsp shallots, chopped
- ✓ 1/2 cup pine nuts, roughly chopped
- ✓ 1/2 cup vegan mayonnaise
- ✓ 1 tbsp deli mustard
- ✓ 2 tbsp fresh basil, chopped
- ✓ 2 tbsp fresh parsley, chopped
- ✓ 1/2 tsp red pepper flakes, crushed
- ✓ Sea salt and freshly ground black pepper, to taste

Directions:

- ❖ Boil the green beans in a large saucepan of salted water until they are just tender or about 2 minutes.
- ❖ Drain and let the beans cool completely; then, transfer them to a salad bowl. Toss the beans with the remaining ingredients.
- ❖ Taste and adjust the seasonings. Enjoy

43) EASY KALE CANNELLINI BEAN SOUP

Preparation Time: 25 minutes | | **Servings: 5**

Ingredients:

- ✓ 1 tbsp olive oil
- ✓ 1/2 tsp ginger, minced
- ✓ 1/2 tsp cumin seeds
- ✓ 1 red onion, chopped
- ✓ 1 carrot, trimmed and chopped
- ✓ 1 parsnip, trimmed and chopped
- ✓ 2 garlic cloves, minced
- ✓ 5 cups vegetable broth
- ✓ 12 ounces Cannellini beans, drained
- ✓ 2 cups kale, torn into pieces
- ✓ Sea salt and ground black pepper, to taste

Directions:

- ❖ In a heavy-bottomed pot, heat the olive over medium-high heat. Now, sauté the ginger and cumin for 1 minute or so.
- ❖ Now, add in the onion, carrot and parsnip; continue sautéing an additional 3 minutes or until the vegetables are just tender.
- ❖ Add in the garlic and continue to sauté for 1 minute or until aromatic.
- ❖ Then, pour in the vegetable broth and bring to a boil. Immediately reduce the heat to a simmer and let it cook for 10 minutes.
- ❖ Fold in the Cannellini beans and kale; continue to simmer until the kale wilts and everything is thoroughly heated. Season with salt and pepper to taste.
- ❖ Ladle into individual bowls and serve hot. Enjoy

44) DELICIOUS MUSHROOM SOUP WITH HEARTY CREAM

Preparation Time: 15 minutes | | **Servings: 5**

Ingredients:

- ✓ 2 tbsp soy butter
- ✓ 1 large shallot, chopped
- ✓ 20 ounces Cremini mushrooms, sliced
- ✓ 2 cloves garlic, minced
- ✓ 4 tbsp flaxseed meal
- ✓ 5 cups vegetable broth
- ✓ 1 1/3 cups full-fat coconut milk
- ✓ 1 bay leaf
- ✓ Sea salt and ground black pepper, to taste

Directions:

- ❖ In a stockpot, melt the vegan butter over medium-high heat. Once hot, cook the shallot for about 3 minutes until tender and fragrant.
- ❖ Add in the mushrooms and garlic and continue cooking until the mushrooms have softened. Add in the flaxseed meal and continue to cook for 1 minute or so.
- ❖ Add in the remaining ingredients. Let it simmer, covered and continue to cook for 5 to 6 minutes more until your soup has thickened slightly.
- ❖ Enjoy

45) ITALIAN-STYLE AUTHENTIC PANZANELLA SALAD

Preparation Time: 35 minutes | | **Servings: 3**

Ingredients:

- ✓ 3 cups artisan bread, broken into 1-inch cubes
- ✓ 3/4-pound asparagus, trimmed and cut into bite-sized pieces
- ✓ 4 tbsp extra-virgin olive oil
- ✓ 1 red onion, chopped
- ✓ 2 tbsp fresh lime juice
- ✓ 1 tsp deli mustard
- ✓ 2 medium heirloom tomatoes, diced
- ✓ 2 cups arugula
- ✓ 2 cups baby spinach
- ✓ 2 Italian peppers, seeded and sliced
- ✓ Sea salt and ground black pepper, to taste

Directions:

- ❖ Arrange the bread cubes on a parchment-lined baking sheet. Bake in the preheated oven at 310 degrees F for about 20 minutes, rotating the baking sheet twice during the baking time; reserve.
- ❖ Turn the oven to 420 degrees F and toss the asparagus with 1 tbsp of olive oil. Roast the asparagus for about 15 minutes or until crisp-tender.
- ❖ Toss the remaining ingredients in a salad bowl; top with the roasted asparagus and toasted bread.
- ❖ Enjoy

Chapter 3. DINNER

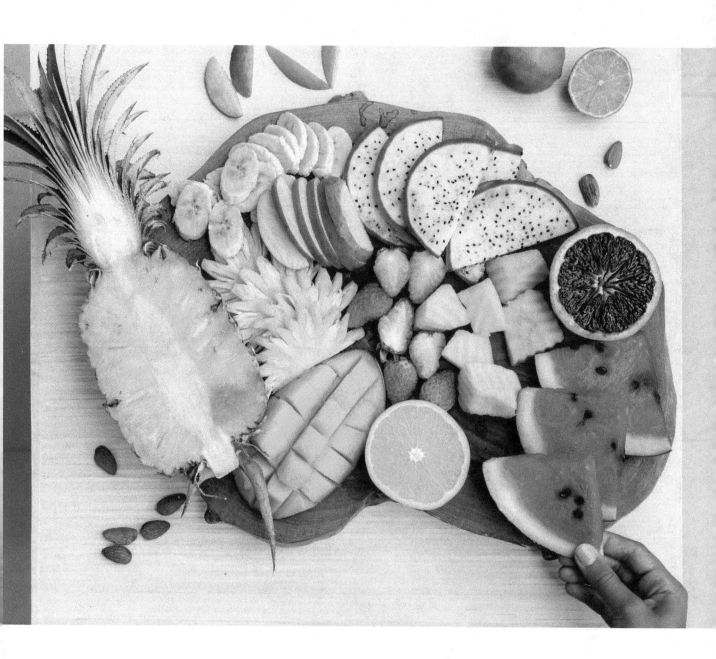

46) ASIAN BLACK BEAN QUINOA SALAD

Preparation Time: 15 minutes + chilling time		Servings: 4

Ingredients:

- ✓ 2 cups water
- ✓ 1 cup quinoa, rinsed
- ✓ 16 ounces canned black beans, drained
- ✓ 2 Roma tomatoes, sliced
- ✓ 1 red onion, thinly sliced
- ✓ 1 cucumber, seeded and chopped
- ✓ 2 cloves garlic, pressed or minced
- ✓ 2 Italian peppers, seeded and sliced
- ✓ 2 tbsp fresh parsley, chopped
- ✓ 2 tbsp fresh cilantro, chopped
- ✓ 1/4 cup olive oil
- ✓ 1 lemon, freshly squeezed
- ✓ 1 tbsp apple cider vinegar
- ✓ 1/2 tsp dried dill weed
- ✓ 1/2 tsp dried oregano
- ✓ Sea salt and ground black pepper, to taste

Directions:

- ❖ Place the water and quinoa in a saucepan and bring it to a rolling boil. Immediately turn the heat to a simmer.
- ❖ Let it simmer for about 13 minutes until the quinoa has absorbed all of the water; fluff the quinoa with a fork and let it cool completely. Then, transfer the quinoa to a salad bowl.
- ❖ Add the remaining ingredients to the salad bowl and toss to combine well. Enjoy

47) MOROCCAN POWER BULGUR SALAD WITH HERBS

Preparation Time: 20 minutes + chilling time		Servings: 4

Ingredients:

- ✓ 2 cups water
- ✓ 1 cup bulgur
- ✓ 12 ounces canned chickpeas, drained
- ✓ 1 Persian cucumber, thinly sliced
- ✓ 2 bell peppers, seeded and thinly sliced
- ✓ 1 jalapeno pepper, seeded and thinly sliced
- ✓ 2 Roma tomatoes, sliced
- ✓ 1 onion, thinly sliced
- ✓ 2 tbsp fresh basil, chopped
- ✓ 2 tbsp fresh parsley, chopped
- ✓ 2 tbsp fresh mint, chopped
- ✓ 2 tbsp fresh chives, chopped
- ✓ 4 tbsp olive oil
- ✓ 1 tbsp balsamic vinegar
- ✓ 1 tbsp lemon juice
- ✓ 1 tsp fresh garlic, pressed
- ✓ Sea salt and freshly ground black pepper, to taste
- ✓ 2 tbsp nutritional yeast
- ✓ 1/2 cup Kalamata olives, sliced

Directions:

- ❖ In a saucepan, bring the water and bulgur to a boil. Immediately turn the heat to a simmer and let it cook for about 20 minutes or until the bulgur is tender and water is almost absorbed. Fluff with a fork and spread on a large tray to let cool.
- ❖ Place the bulgur in a salad bowl followed by the chickpeas, cucumber, peppers, tomatoes, onion, basil, parsley, mint and chives.
- ❖ In a small mixing dish, whisk the olive oil, balsamic vinegar, lemon juice, garlic, salt and black pepper. Dress the salad and toss to combine.
- ❖ Sprinkle nutritional yeast over the top, garnish with olives and serve at room temperature. Enjoy

48) AUTHENTIC ROASTED PEPPER SALAD

Preparation Time: 15 minutes + chilling time		Servings: 3

Ingredients:

- ✓ 6 bell peppers
- ✓ 3 tbsp extra-virgin olive oil
- ✓ 3 tsp red wine vinegar
- ✓ 3 garlic cloves, finely chopped
- ✓ 2 tbsp fresh parsley, chopped
- ✓ Sea salt and freshly cracked black pepper, to taste
- ✓ 1/2 tsp red pepper flakes
- ✓ 6 tbsp pine nuts, roughly chopped

Directions:

- ❖ Broil the peppers on a parchment-lined baking sheet for about 10 minutes, rotating the pan halfway through the cooking time, until they are charred on all sides.
- ❖ Then, cover the peppers with a plastic wrap to steam. Discard the skin, seeds and cores.
- ❖ Slice the peppers into strips and toss them with the remaining ingredients. Place in your refrigerator until ready to serve. Enjoy

49) AUTUMN HEARTY QUINOA SOUP

Preparation Time: 25 minutes | | **Servings: 4**

Ingredients:

- ✓ 2 tbsp olive oil
- ✓ 1 onion, chopped
- ✓ 2 carrots, peeled and chopped
- ✓ 1 parsnip, chopped
- ✓ 1 celery stalk, chopped
- ✓ 1 cup yellow squash, chopped
- ✓ 4 garlic cloves, pressed or minced

- ✓ 4 cups roasted vegetable broth
- ✓ 2 medium tomatoes, crushed
- ✓ 1 cup quinoa
- ✓ Sea salt and ground black pepper, to taste
- ✓ 1 bay laurel
- ✓ 2 cup Swiss chard, tough ribs removed and torn into pieces
- ✓ 2 tbsp Italian parsley, chopped

Directions:

- ❖ In a heavy-bottomed pot, heat the olive over medium-high heat. Now, sauté the onion, carrot, parsnip, celery and yellow squash for about 3 minutes or until the vegetables are just tender.
- ❖ Add in the garlic and continue to sauté for 1 minute or until aromatic.
- ❖ Then, stir in the vegetable broth, tomatoes, quinoa, salt, pepper and bay laurel; bring to a boil. Immediately reduce the heat to a simmer and let it cook for 13 minutes.
- ❖ Fold in the Swiss chard; continue to simmer until the chard wilts.
- ❖ Ladle into individual bowls and serve garnished with the fresh parsley. Enjoy

50) SPECIAL GREEN LENTIL SALAD

Preparation Time: 20 minutes + chilling time | | **Servings: 5**

Ingredients:

- ✓ 1 ½ cups green lentils, rinsed
- ✓ 2 cups arugula
- ✓ 2 cups Romaine lettuce, torn into pieces
- ✓ 1 cup baby spinach
- ✓ 1/4 cup fresh basil, chopped
- ✓ 1/2 cup shallots, chopped

- ✓ 2 garlic cloves, finely chopped
- ✓ 1/4 cup oil-packed sun-dried tomatoes, rinsed and chopped
- ✓ 5 tbsp extra-virgin olive oil
- ✓ 3 tbsp fresh lemon juice
- ✓ Sea salt and ground black pepper, to taste

Directions:

- ❖ In a large-sized saucepan, bring 4 ½ cups of the water and red lentils to a boil.
- ❖ Immediately turn the heat to a simmer and continue to cook your lentils for a further 15 to 17 minutes or until they've softened but not mushy. Drain and let it cool completely.
- ❖ Transfer the lentils to a salad bowl; toss the lentils with the remaining ingredients until well combined.
- ❖ Serve chilled or at room temperature. Enjoy

51) EASY CHICKPEA, ACORN SQUASH, AND COUSCOUS SOUP

Preparation Time: 20 minutes | | **Servings: 4**

Ingredients:

- ✓ 2 tbsp olive oil
- ✓ 1 shallot, chopped
- ✓ 1 carrot, trimmed and chopped
- ✓ 2 cups acorn squash, chopped
- ✓ 1 stalk celery, chopped
- ✓ 1 tsp garlic, finely chopped
- ✓ 1 tsp dried rosemary, chopped
- ✓ 1 tsp dried thyme, chopped

- ✓ 2 cups cream of onion soup
- ✓ 2 cups water
- ✓ 1 cup dry couscous
- ✓ Sea salt and ground black pepper, to taste
- ✓ 1/2 tsp red pepper flakes
- ✓ 6 ounces canned chickpeas, drained
- ✓ 2 tbsp fresh lemon juice

Directions:

- ❖ In a heavy-bottomed pot, heat the olive over medium-high heat. Now, sauté the shallot, carrot, acorn squash and celery for about 3 minutes or until the vegetables are just tender.
- ❖ Add in the garlic, rosemary and thyme and continue to sauté for 1 minute or until aromatic.
- ❖ Then, stir in the soup, water, couscous, salt, black pepper and red pepper flakes; bring to a boil. Immediately reduce the heat to a simmer and let it cook for 12 minutes.
- ❖ Fold in the canned chickpeas; continue to simmer until heated through or about 5 minutes more.
- ❖ Ladle into individual bowls and drizzle with the lemon juice over the top. Enjoy

52) DELICIOUS GARLIC CROSTINI WITH CABBAGE SOUP

Preparation Time: 1 hour		Servings: 4

Ingredients:

- ✓ Soup:
- ✓ 2 tbsp olive oil
- ✓ 1 medium leek, chopped
- ✓ 1 cup turnip, chopped
- ✓ 1 parsnip, chopped
- ✓ 1 carrot, chopped
- ✓ 2 cups cabbage, shredded
- ✓ 2 garlic cloves, finely chopped
- ✓ 4 cups vegetable broth

- ✓ 2 bay leaves
- ✓ Sea salt and ground black pepper, to taste
- ✓ 1/4 tsp cumin seeds
- ✓ 1/2 tsp mustard seeds
- ✓ 1 tsp dried basil
- ✓ 2 tomatoes, pureed
- ✓ Crostini:
- ✓ 8 slices of baguette
- ✓ 2 heads garlic
- ✓ 4 tbsp extra-virgin olive oil

Directions:

- ❖ In a soup pot, heat 2 tbsp of the olive over medium-high heat. Now, sauté the leek, turnip, parsnip and carrot for about 4 minutes or until the vegetables are crisp-tender.
- ❖ Add in the garlic and cabbage and continue to sauté for 1 minute or until aromatic.
- ❖ Then, stir in the vegetable broth, bay leaves, salt, black pepper, cumin seeds, mustard seeds, dried basil and pureed tomatoes; bring to a boil. Immediately reduce the heat to a simmer and let it cook for about 20 minutes.
- ❖ Meanwhile, preheat your oven to 375 degrees F. Now, roast the garlic and baguette slices for about 15 minutes. Remove the crostini from the oven.
- ❖ Continue baking the garlic for 45 minutes more or until very tender. Allow the garlic to cool.
- ❖ Now, cut each head of the garlic using a sharp serrated knife in order to separate all the cloves.
- ❖ Squeeze the roasted garlic cloves out of their skins. Mash the garlic pulp with 4 tbsp of the extra-virgin olive oil.
- ❖ Spread the roasted garlic mixture evenly on the tops of the crostini. Serve with the warm soup. Enjoy

53) TASTY GREEN BEAN SOUP CREAM

Preparation Time: 35 minutes		Servings: 4

Ingredients:

- ✓ 1 tbsp sesame oil
- ✓ 1 onion, chopped
- ✓ 1 green pepper, seeded and chopped
- ✓ 2 russet potatoes, peeled and diced
- ✓ 2 garlic cloves, chopped

- ✓ 4 cups vegetable broth
- ✓ 1 pound green beans, trimmed
- ✓ Sea salt and ground black pepper, to season
- ✓ 1 cup full-fat coconut milk

Directions:

- ❖ In a heavy-bottomed pot, heat the sesame over medium-high heat. Now, sauté the onion, peppers and potatoes for about 5 minutes, stirring periodically.
- ❖ Add in the garlic and continue sautéing for 1 minute or until fragrant.
- ❖ Then, stir in the vegetable broth, green beans, salt and black pepper; bring to a boil. Immediately reduce the heat to a simmer and let it cook for 20 minutes.
- ❖ Puree the green bean mixture using an immersion blender until creamy and uniform.
- ❖ Return the pureed mixture to the pot. Fold in the coconut milk and continue to simmer until heated through or about 5 minutes longer.
- ❖ Ladle into individual bowls and serve hot. Enjoy

54) FRENCH ORIGINAL ONION SOUP

Preparation Time: 1 hour 30 minutes

Servings: 4

Ingredients:

- ✓ 2 tbsp olive oil
- ✓ 2 large yellow onions, thinly sliced
- ✓ 2 thyme sprigs, chopped
- ✓ 2 rosemary sprigs, chopped
- ✓ 2 tsp balsamic vinegar
- ✓ 4 cups vegetable stock
- ✓ Sea salt and ground black pepper, to taste

Directions:

- ❖ In a or Dutch oven, heat the olive oil over a moderate heat. Now, cook the onions with thyme, rosemary and 1 tsp of the sea salt for about 2 minutes.
- ❖ Now, turn the heat to medium-low and continue cooking until the onions caramelize or about 50 minutes.
- ❖ Add in the balsamic vinegar and continue to cook for a further 15 more. Add in the stock, salt and black pepper and continue simmering for 20 to 25 minutes.
- ❖ Serve with toasted bread and enjoy

55) SUPER ROASTED CARROT SOUP

Preparation Time: 50 minutes

Servings: 4

Ingredients:

- ✓ 1 ½ pounds carrots
- ✓ 4 tbsp olive oil
- ✓ 1 yellow onion, chopped
- ✓ 2 cloves garlic, minced
- ✓ 1/3 tsp ground cumin
- ✓ Sea salt and white pepper, to taste
- ✓ 1/2 tsp turmeric powder
- ✓ 4 cups vegetable stock
- ✓ 2 tsp lemon juice
- ✓ 2 tbsp fresh cilantro, roughly chopped

Directions:

- ❖ Start by preheating your oven to 400 degrees F. Place the carrots on a large parchment-lined baking sheet; toss the carrots with 2 tbsp of the olive oil.
- ❖ Roast the carrots for about 35 minutes or until they've softened.
- ❖ In a heavy-bottomed pot, heat the remaining 2 tbsp of the olive oil. Now, sauté the onion and garlic for about 3 minutes or until aromatic.
- ❖ Add in the cumin, salt, pepper, turmeric, vegetable stock and roasted carrots. Continue to simmer for 12 minutes more.
- ❖ Puree your soup with an immersion blender. Drizzle lemon juice over your soup and serve garnished with fresh cilantro leaves. Enjoy

56) ITALIAN-STYLE PENNE PASTA SALAD

Preparation Time: 15 minutes + chilling time

Servings: 3

Ingredients:

- ✓ 9 ounces penne pasta
- ✓ 9 ounces canned Cannellini bean, drained
- ✓ 1 small onion, thinly sliced
- ✓ 1/3 cup Niçoise olives, pitted and sliced
- ✓ 2 Italian peppers, sliced
- ✓ 1 cup cherry tomatoes, halved
- ✓ 3 cups arugula
- ✓ Dressing:
- ✓ 3 tbsp extra-virgin olive oil
- ✓ 1 tsp lemon zest
- ✓ 1 tsp garlic, minced
- ✓ 3 tbsp balsamic vinegar
- ✓ 1 tsp Italian herb mix
- ✓ Sea salt and ground black pepper, to taste

Directions:

- ❖ Cook the penne pasta according to the package directions. Drain and rinse the pasta. Let it cool completely and then, transfer it to a salad bowl.
- ❖ Then, add the beans, onion, olives, peppers, tomatoes and arugula to the salad bowl.
- ❖ Mix all the dressing ingredients until everything is well incorporated. Dress your salad and serve well

57) SPECIAL CHANA CHAAT INDIAN SALAD

Preparation Time: 45 minutes + chilling time		Servings: 4

Ingredients:

- ✓ 1 pound dry chickpeas, soaked overnight
- ✓ 2 San Marzano tomatoes, diced
- ✓ 1 Persian cucumber, sliced
- ✓ 1 onion, chopped
- ✓ 1 bell pepper, seeded and thinly sliced
- ✓ 1 green chili, seeded and thinly sliced
- ✓ 2 handfuls baby spinach
- ✓ 1/2 tsp Kashmiri chili powder
- ✓ 4 curry leaves, chopped
- ✓ 1 tbsp chaat masala
- ✓ 2 tbsp fresh lemon juice, or to taste
- ✓ 4 tbsp olive oil
- ✓ 1 tsp agave syrup
- ✓ 1/2 tsp mustard seeds
- ✓ 1/2 tsp coriander seeds
- ✓ 2 tbsp sesame seeds, lightly toasted
- ✓ 2 tbsp fresh cilantro, roughly chopped

Directions:

- ❖ Drain the chickpeas and transfer them to a large saucepan. Cover the chickpeas with water by 2 inches and bring it to a boil.
- ❖ Immediately turn the heat to a simmer and continue to cook for approximately 40 minutes.
- ❖ Toss the chickpeas with the tomatoes, cucumber, onion, peppers, spinach, chili powder, curry leaves and chaat masala.
- ❖ In a small mixing dish, thoroughly combine the lemon juice, olive oil, agave syrup, mustard seeds and coriander seeds.
- ❖ Garnish with sesame seeds and fresh cilantro. Enjoy

58) ORIGINAL TEMPEH AND NOODLE SALAD THAI-STYLE

Preparation Time: 45 minutes		Servings: 3

Ingredients:

- ✓ 6 ounces tempeh
- ✓ 4 tbsp rice vinegar
- ✓ 4 tbsp soy sauce
- ✓ 2 garlic cloves, minced
- ✓ 1 small-sized lime, freshly juiced
- ✓ 5 ounces rice noodles
- ✓ 1 carrot, julienned
- ✓ 1 shallot, chopped
- ✓ 3 handfuls Chinese cabbage, thinly sliced
- ✓ 3 handfuls kale, torn into pieces
- ✓ 1 bell pepper, seeded and thinly sliced
- ✓ 1 bird's eye chili, minced
- ✓ 1/4 cup peanut butter
- ✓ 2 tbsp agave syrup

Directions:

- ❖ Place the tempeh, 2 tbsp of the rice vinegar, soy sauce, garlic and lime juice in a ceramic dish; let it marinate for about 40 minutes.
- ❖ Meanwhile, cook the rice noodles according to the package directions. Drain your noodles and transfer them to a salad bowl.
- ❖ Add the carrot, shallot, cabbage, kale and peppers to the salad bowl. Add in the peanut butter, the remaining 2 tbsp of the rice vinegar and agave syrup and toss to combine well.
- ❖ Top with the marinated tempeh and serve immediately. Enjoy

59) TYPICAL CREAM OF BROCCOLI SOUP

Preparation Time: 35 minutes		Servings: 4

Ingredients:

- ✓ 2 tbsp olive oil
- ✓ 1 pound broccoli florets
- ✓ 1 onion, chopped
- ✓ 1 celery rib, chopped
- ✓ 1 parsnip, chopped
- ✓ 1 tsp garlic, chopped
- ✓ 3 cups vegetable broth
- ✓ 1/2 tsp dried dill
- ✓ 1/2 tsp dried oregano
- ✓ Sea salt and ground black pepper, to taste
- ✓ 2 tbsp flaxseed meal
- ✓ 1 cup full-fat coconut milk

Directions:

- ❖ In a heavy-bottomed pot, heat the olive oil over medium-high heat. Now, sauté the broccoli onion, celery and parsnip for about 5 minutes, stirring periodically.
- ❖ Add in the garlic and continue sautéing for 1 minute or until fragrant.
- ❖ Then, stir in the vegetable broth, dill, oregano, salt and black pepper; bring to a boil. Immediately reduce the heat to a simmer and let it cook for about 20 minutes.
- ❖ Puree the soup using an immersion blender until creamy and uniform.
- ❖ Return the pureed mixture to the pot. Fold in the flaxseed meal and coconut milk; continue to simmer until heated through or about 5 minutes.
- ❖ Ladle into four serving bowls and enjoy

60) EASY RAISIN MOROCCAN LENTIL SALAD

Preparation Time: 20 minutes + chilling time | | **Servings:** 4

Ingredients:

- ✓ 1 cup red lentils, rinsed
- ✓ 1 large carrot, julienned
- ✓ 1 Persian cucumber, thinly sliced
- ✓ 1 sweet onion, chopped
- ✓ 1/2 cup golden raisins
- ✓ 1/4 cup fresh mint, snipped
- ✓ 1/4 cup fresh basil, snipped
- ✓ 1/4 cup extra-virgin olive oil
- ✓ 1/4 cup lemon juice, freshly squeezed
- ✓ 1 tsp grated lemon peel
- ✓ 1/2 tsp fresh ginger root, peeled and minced
- ✓ 1/2 tsp granulated garlic
- ✓ 1 tsp ground allspice
- ✓ Sea salt and ground black pepper, to taste

Directions:

- ❖ In a large-sized saucepan, bring 3 cups of the water and 1 cup of the lentils to a boil.
- ❖ Immediately turn the heat to a simmer and continue to cook your lentils for a further 15 to 17 minutes or until they've softened but are not mushy yet. Drain and let it cool completely.
- ❖ Transfer the lentils to a salad bowl; add in the carrot, cucumber and sweet onion. Then, add the raisins, mint and basil to your salad.
- ❖ In a small mixing dish, whisk the olive oil, lemon juice, lemon peel, ginger, granulated garlic, allspice, salt and black pepper.
- ❖ Dress your salad and serve well-chilled. Enjoy

61) RICH CHICKPEA AND ASPARAGUS SALAD

Preparation Time: 10 minutes + chilling time | | **Servings:** 5

Ingredients:

- ✓ 1 ¼ pounds asparagus, trimmed and cut into bite-sized pieces
- ✓ 5 ounces canned chickpeas, drained and rinsed
- ✓ 1 chipotle pepper, seeded and chopped
- ✓ 1 Italian pepper, seeded and chopped
- ✓ 1/4 cup fresh basil leaves, chopped
- ✓ 1/4 cup fresh parsley leaves, chopped
- ✓ 2 tbsp fresh mint leaves
- ✓ 2 tbsp fresh chives, chopped
- ✓ 1 tsp garlic, minced
- ✓ 1/4 cup extra-virgin olive oil
- ✓ 1 tbsp balsamic vinegar
- ✓ 1 tbsp fresh lime juice
- ✓ 2 tbsp soy sauce
- ✓ 1/4 tsp ground allspice
- ✓ 1/4 tsp ground cumin
- ✓ Sea salt and freshly cracked peppercorns, to taste

Directions:

- ❖ Bring a large pot of salted water with the asparagus to a boil; let it cook for 2 minutes; drain and rinse.
- ❖ Transfer the asparagus to a salad bowl.
- ❖ Toss the asparagus with the chickpeas, peppers, herbs, garlic, olive oil, vinegar, lime juice, soy sauce and spices.
- ❖ Toss to combine and serve immediately. Enjoy

62) OLD-FASHIONED GREEK GREEN BEAN SALAD

Preparation Time: 10 minutes + chilling time | | **Servings:** 4

Ingredients:

- ✓ 1 ½ pounds green beans, trimmed
- ✓ 1/2 cup scallions, chopped
- ✓ 1 tsp garlic, minced
- ✓ 1 Persian cucumber, sliced
- ✓ 2 cups grape tomatoes, halved
- ✓ 1/4 cup olive oil
- ✓ 1 tsp deli mustard
- ✓ 2 tbsp tamari sauce
- ✓ 2 tbsp lemon juice
- ✓ 1 tbsp apple cider vinegar
- ✓ 1/4 tsp cumin powder
- ✓ 1/2 tsp dried thyme
- ✓ Sea salt and ground black pepper, to taste

Directions:

- ❖ Boil the green beans in a large saucepan of salted water until they are just tender or about 2 minutes.
- ❖ Drain and let the beans cool completely; then, transfer them to a salad bowl. Toss the beans with the remaining ingredients.
- ❖ Enjoy

63) AUTUMN BEAN SOUP

Preparation Time: 25 minutes		Servings: 4

Ingredients:

- ✓ 1 tbsp olive oil
- ✓ 2 tbsp shallots, chopped
- ✓ 1 carrot, chopped
- ✓ 1 parsnip, chopped
- ✓ 1 celery stalk, chopped
- ✓ 1 tsp fresh garlic, minced
- ✓ 4 cups vegetable broth
- ✓ 2 bay leaves
- ✓ 1 rosemary sprig, chopped
- ✓ 16 ounces canned navy beans
- ✓ Flaky sea salt and ground black pepper, to taste

Directions:

- ❖ In a heavy-bottomed pot, heat the olive over medium-high heat. Now, sauté the shallots, carrot, parsnip and celery for approximately 3 minutes or until the vegetables are just tender.
- ❖ Add in the garlic and continue to sauté for 1 minute or until aromatic.
- ❖ Then, add in the vegetable broth, bay leaves and rosemary and bring to a boil. Immediately reduce the heat to a simmer and let it cook for 10 minutes.
- ❖ Fold in the navy beans and continue to simmer for about 5 minutes longer until everything is thoroughly heated. Season with salt and black pepper to taste.
- ❖ Ladle into individual bowls, discard the bay leaves and serve hot. Enjoy

64) ITALIAN CREAM MUSHROOMS SOUP

Preparation Time: 15 minutes		Servings: 3

Ingredients:

- ✓ 3 tbsp vegan butter
- ✓ 1 white onion, chopped
- ✓ 1 red bell pepper, chopped
- ✓ 1/2 tsp garlic, pressed
- ✓ 3 cups Cremini mushrooms, chopped
- ✓ 2 tbsp almond flour
- ✓ 3 cups water
- ✓ 1 tsp Italian herb mix
- ✓ Sea salt and ground black pepper, to taste
- ✓ 1 heaping tbsp fresh chives, roughly chopped

Directions:

- ❖ In a stockpot, melt the vegan butter over medium-high heat. Once hot, sauté the onion and pepper for about 3 minutes until they have softened.
- ❖ Add in the garlic and Cremini mushrooms and continue sautéing until the mushrooms have softened. Sprinkle almond meal over the mushrooms and continue to cook for 1 minute or so.
- ❖ Add in the remaining ingredients. Let it simmer, covered and continue to cook for 5 to 6 minutes more until the liquid has thickened slightly.
- ❖ Ladle into three soup bowls and garnish with fresh chives. Enjoy

65) TASTY ROASTED BASIL AND TOMATO SOUP

Preparation Time: 60 minutes		Servings: 4

Ingredients:

- ✓ 2 lb tomatoes, halved
- ✓ 2 tsp garlic powder
- ✓ 3 tbsp olive oil
- ✓ 1 tbsp balsamic vinegar
- ✓ Salt and black pepper to taste
- ✓ 4 shallots, chopped
- ✓ 2 cups vegetable broth
- ✓ ½ cup basil leaves, chopped

Directions:

- ❖ Preheat oven to 450 F.
- ❖ In a bowl, mix tomatoes, garlic, 2 tbsp of oil, vinegar, salt, and pepper. Arrange the tomatoes onto a baking dish. Sprinkle with some olive oil, garlic powder, balsamic vinegar, salt, and pepper. Bake for 30 minutes until the tomatoes get dark brown color. Take out from the oven; reserve.
- ❖ Heat the remaining oil in a pot over medium heat. Place the shallots and cook for 3 minutes, stirring often. Add in roasted tomatoes and broth. Bring to a boil, then lower the heat and simmer for 10 minutes. Transfer to a food processor and blitz the soup until smooth. Serve topped with basil

33

66) SPECIAL UNDER PRESSURE COOKER GREEN ONION AND POTATO SOUP

Preparation Time: 25 minutes | | **Servings: 5**

Ingredients:

- ✓ 3 green onions, chopped
- ✓ 4 garlic cloves, minced
- ✓ 1 tbsp olive oil
- ✓ 6 russet potatoes, chopped

- ✓ ½ (13.5-oz) can coconut milk
- ✓ 5 cups vegetable broth
- ✓ Salt and black pepper to taste

Directions:

- ❖ Set your IP to Sauté. Place in green onions, garlic, and olive oil. Cook for 3 minutes until softened. Add in potatoes, coconut milk, broth, and salt. Lock the lid in place, set time to 6 minutes on High. Once ready, perform a natural pressure release for 10 minutes. Allow cooling for a few minutes. Using an immersion blender, blitz the soup until smooth. Serve

67) EASY AND QUICK BELL PEPPER AND MUSHROOM SOUP

Preparation Time: 45 minutes | | **Servings: 6**

Ingredients:

- ✓ 3 tbsp olive oil
- ✓ 1 onion, chopped
- ✓ 1 large carrot, chopped
- ✓ 1 lb mixed bell peppers, chopped
- ✓ 1 cup cremini mushrooms, quartered

- ✓ 1 cup white mushrooms, quartered
- ✓ 6 cups vegetable broth
- ✓ ¼ cup chopped fresh parsley
- ✓ 1 tsp minced fresh thyme
- ✓ Salt and black pepper to taste

Directions:

- ❖ Heat the oil in a pot over medium heat. Place onion, carrot, and celery and cook for 5 minutes. Add in bell peppers and broth and stir. Bring to a boil, lower the heat, and simmer for 20 minutes. Adjust the seasoning with salt and black pepper. Serve in soup bowls topped with parsley and thyme

68) SPECIAL PUMPKIN CAYENNE SOUP

Preparation Time: 55 minutes | | **Servings: 6**

Ingredients:

- ✓ 1 (2-pound) pumpkin, sliced
- ✓ 3 tbsp olive oil
- ✓ 1 tsp salt
- ✓ 2 red bell peppers
- ✓ 1 onion, halved
- ✓ 1 head garlic

- ✓ 6 cups water
- ✓ Zest and juice of 1 lime
- ✓ ¼ tsp cayenne pepper
- ✓ ½ tsp ground coriander
- ✓ ½ tsp ground cumin
- ✓ Toasted pumpkin seeds

Directions:

- ❖ Preheat oven to 350 F.
- ❖ Brush the pumpkin slices with oil and sprinkle with salt. Arrange the slices skin-side-down and on a greased baking dish and bake for 20 minutes. Brush the onion with oil. Cut the top of the garlic head and brush with oil.
- ❖ When the pumpkin is ready, add in bell peppers, onion, and garlic, and bake for another 10 minutes. Allow cooling.
- ❖ Take out the flesh from the pumpkin skin and transfer to a food processor. Cut the pepper roughly, peel and cut the onion, and remove the cloves from the garlic head. Transfer to the food processor and pour in the water, lime zest, and lime juice.
- ❖ Blend the soup until smooth. If it's very thick, add a bit of water to reach your desired consistency. Sprinkle with salt, cayenne, coriander, and cumin. Serve

69) EASY ZUCCHINI CREAM SOUP WITH WALNUTS

Preparation Time: 45 minutes		Servings: 4

Ingredients:

- ✓ 3 zucchinis, chopped
- ✓ 2 tsp olive oil
- ✓ Sea salt and black pepper to taste
- ✓ 1 onion, diced
- ✓ 4 cups vegetable stock
- ✓ 3 tsp ground sage
- ✓ 3 tbsp nutritional yeast
- ✓ 1 cup non-dairy milk
- ✓ ¼ cup toasted walnuts

Directions:

❖ Heat the oil in a skillet and place zucchini, onion, salt, and pepper; cook for 5 minutes. Pour in vegetable stock and bring to a boil. Lower the heat and simmer for 15 minutes. Stir in sage, nutritional yeast, and milk. Purée the soup with a blender until smooth. Serve garnished with toasted walnuts and pepper

70) TRADITIONAL RAMEN SOUP

Preparation Time: 25 minutes		Servings: 4

Ingredients:

- ✓ 7 oz Japanese buckwheat noodles
- ✓ 4 tbsp sesame paste
- ✓ 1 cup canned pinto beans, drained
- ✓ 2 tbsp fresh cilantro, chopped
- ✓ 2 scallions, thinly sliced

Directions:

❖ In boiling salted water, add in the noodles and cook for 5 minutes over low heat. Remove a cup of the noodle water to a bowl and add in the sesame paste; stir until it has dissolved. Pour the sesame mix in the pot with the noodles, add in pinto beans, and stir until everything is hot. Serve topped with cilantro and scallions in individual bowls

71) MEXICAN BLACK-EYED PEA SOUP

Preparation Time: 45 minutes		Servings: 6

Ingredients:

- ✓ 2 carrots, chopped
- ✓ 1 onion, chopped
- ✓ 2 cups canned dried black-eyed peas
- ✓ 1 tbsp soy sauce
- ✓ 3 tsp dried thyme
- ✓ 1 tsp onion powder
- ✓ ½ tsp garlic powder
- ✓ Salt and black pepper to taste
- ✓ ¼ cup chopped pitted black olives

Directions:

❖ Place carrots, onion, black-eyed peas, 3 cups water, soy sauce, thyme, onion powder, garlic powder, and pepper in a pot. Bring to a boil, then reduce the heat to low. Cook for 20 minutes. Allow cooling for a few minutes. Transfer to a food processor and blend until smooth. Stir in black olives. Serve

Chapter 4. DESSERTS

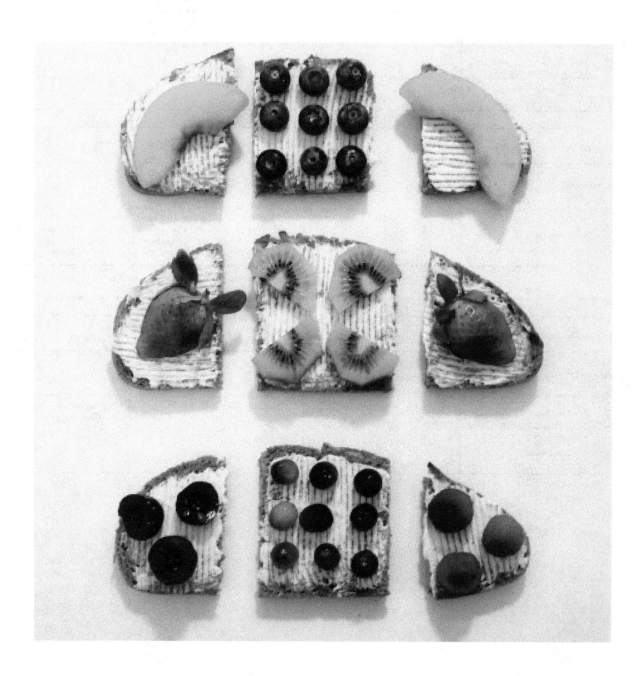

72) ITALIAN BERRY MACEDONIA WITH MINT

Preparation Time: 20 minutes		Servings: 4

Ingredients:

- ✓ ¼ cup lemon juice
- ✓ 4 tsp agave syrup
- ✓ 2 cups chopped pears
- ✓ 2 cups chopped strawberries
- ✓ 3 cups mixed berries
- ✓ 8 fresh mint leaves

Directions:

- ❖ Chop half of the mint leaves; reserve.
- ❖ In a large bowl, combine together pears, strawberries, raspberries, blackberries, and half of the mint leaves. Divide the Macedonia salad between 4 small cups. Top with lemon juice, agave syrup, and mint leaves and serve chilled

73) SPECIAL CINNAMON PUMPKIN PIE

Preparation Time: 1 hr 10 min + cooling time		Servings: 4

Ingredients:

- ✓ For the piecrust:
- ✓ 4 tbsp flaxseed powder
- ✓ 1/3 cup whole-wheat flour
- ✓ ½ tsp salt
- ✓ ¼ cup cold plant butter, crumbled
- ✓ 3 tbsp pure malt syrup
- ✓ For the filling:
- ✓ 2 tbsp flaxseed powder + 6 tbsp water
- ✓ 4 tbsp plant butter
- ✓ ¼ cup pure maple syrup
- ✓ ¼ cup pure date sugar
- ✓ 1 tsp cinnamon powder
- ✓ ½ tsp ginger powder
- ✓ 1/8 tsp cloves powder
- ✓ 1 (15 oz) can pumpkin purée
- ✓ 1 cup almond milk

Directions:

- ❖ Preheat oven to 350 F. In a bowl, mix flaxseed powder with 12 tbsp water and allow thickening for 5 minutes. Do this for the filling's vegan "flax egg" too in another bowl. In a bowl, combine flour and salt. Add in plant butter and whisk until crumbly. Pour in crust's vegan "flax egg," maple syrup, vanilla, and mix until smooth dough forms. Flatten, cover with plastic wrap, and refrigerate for 1 hour.
- ❖ Dust a working surface with flour, remove the dough onto the surface and flatten it into a 1-inch diameter circle. Lay the dough on a greased pie pan and press to fit the shape of the pan. Use a knife to trim the edges of the pan. Lay a parchment paper on the dough, pour on some baking beans and bake for 15-20 minutes. Remove, pour out the baking beans, and allow cooling. In a bowl, whisk filling's flaxseed, butter, maple syrup, date sugar, cinnamon powder, ginger powder, cloves powder, pumpkin puree, and almond milk. Pour the mixture onto the piecrust and bake for 35-40 minutes

74) EVERYTIME PARTY MATCHA AND HAZELNUT CHEESECAKE

Preparation Time: 20 minutes + cooling time		Servings: 4

Ingredients:

- ✓ 2/3 cup toasted rolled oats
- ✓ ¼ cup plant butter, melted
- ✓ 3 tbsp pure date sugar
- ✓ 6 oz cashew cream cheese
- ✓ ¼ cup almond milk
- ✓ 1 tbsp matcha powder
- ✓ ¼ cup just-boiled water
- ✓ 3 tsp agar agar powder
- ✓ 2 tbsp toasted hazelnuts, chopped

Directions:

- ❖ Process the oats, butter, and date sugar in a blender until smooth.
- ❖ Pour the mixture into a greased 9-inch springform pan and press the mixture onto the bottom of the pan. Refrigerate for 30 minutes until firm while you make the filling.
- ❖ In a large bowl, using an electric mixer, whisk the cashew cream cheese until smooth. Beat in the almond milk and mix in the matcha powder until smooth.
- ❖ Mix the boiled water and agar agar until dissolved and whisk this mixture into the creamy mix. Fold in the hazelnuts until well distributed. Remove the cake pan from the fridge and pour in the cream mixture. Shake the pan to ensure a smooth layering on top. Refrigerate further for at least 3 hours. Take out the cake pan, release the cake, slice, and serve

75) ITALIAN PISTACHIOS AND CHOCOLATE POPSICLES

Preparation Time: 5 minutes + cooling time | | **Servings:** 4

Ingredients:

- ✓ ½ cup chocolate chips, melted
- ✓ 1 ½ cups oat milk
- ✓ 1 tbsp unsweetened cocoa powder
- ✓ 3 tbsp pure date syrup
- ✓ 1 tsp vanilla extract
- ✓ A handful of pistachios, chopped

Directions:

- ❖ In a blender, add chocolate, oat milk, cocoa powder, date syrup, vanilla, pistachios, and process until smooth. Divide the mixture into popsicle molds and freeze for 3 hours. Dip the popsicle molds in warm water to loosen the popsicles and pull out the popsicles

76) ENGLISH OATMEAL COOKIES WITH HAZELNUTS

Preparation Time: 15 minutes | | **Servings:** 2

Ingredients:

- ✓ 1 ½ cups whole-grain flour
- ✓ 1 tsp baking powder
- ✓ ⅛ tsp salt
- ✓ 1 tsp ground cinnamon
- ✓ ¼ tsp ground nutmeg
- ✓ 1 ½ cups old-fashioned oats
- ✓ 1 cup chopped hazelnuts
- ✓ ½ cup plant butter, melted
- ✓ ½ cup pure maple syrup
- ✓ ¼ cup pure date sugar
- ✓ 2 tsp pure vanilla extract

Directions:

- ❖ Preheat oven to 360 F.
- ❖ Combine the flour, baking powder, salt, cinnamon, and nutmeg in a bowl. Add in oats and hazelnuts. In another bowl, whisk the butter, maple syrup, sugar, and vanilla. Pour over the flour mixture. Mix well. Spoon a small ball of cookie dough on a baking sheet and press down with a fork. Bake for 10-12 minutes, until browned. Let completely cool on a rack

77) TROPICAL COCONUT CHOCOLATE TRUFFLES

Preparation Time: 1 hour 15 minutes | | **Servings:** 12

Ingredients:

- ✓ 1 cup raw cashews, soaked overnight
- ✓ ¾ cup pitted cherries
- ✓ 2 tbsp coconut oil
- ✓ 1 cup shredded coconut
- ✓ 2 tbsp cocoa powder

Directions:

- ❖ Line a baking sheet with parchment paper and set aside.
- ❖ Blend cashews, cherries, coconut oil, half of the shredded coconut, and cocoa powder in a food processor until ingredients are evenly mixed. Spread the remaining shredded coconut on a dish. Mold the mixture into 12 truffle shapes. Roll the truffles in the coconut dish, shaking off any excess, then arrange on the prepared baking sheet. Refrigerate for 1 hour

78) DELICIOUS LAYERED RASPBERRY AND TOFU CUPS

Preparation Time: 60 minutes		Servings: 4

Ingredients:

- ✓ ½ cup unsalted raw cashews
- ✓ 3 tbsp pure date sugar
- ✓ ½ cup soy milk
- ✓ ¾ cup firm silken tofu, drained
- ✓ 1 tsp vanilla extract
- ✓ 2 cups sliced raspberries
- ✓ 1 tsp fresh lemon juice
- ✓ Fresh mint leaves

Directions:

- ❖ Grind the cashews and 3 tbsp of date sugar in a blender until a fine powder is obtained. Pour in soy milk and blitz until smooth. Add in tofu and vanilla and pulse until creamy. Remove to a bowl and refrigerate covered for 30 minutes.
- ❖ In a bowl, mix the raspberries, lemon juice, and remaining date sugar. Let sit for 20 minutes. Assemble by alternating into small cups, one layer of raspberries and one layer of cashew cream, ending with the cashew cream. Serve garnished with mint leaves

79) EASY CASHEW AND CRANBERRY TRUFFLES

Preparation Time: 15 minutes		Servings: 4

Ingredients:

- ✓ 2 cups fresh cranberries
- ✓ 2 tbsp pure date syrup
- ✓ 1 tsp vanilla extract
- ✓ 16 oz cashew cream
- ✓ 4 tbsp plant butter
- ✓ 3 tbsp unsweetened cocoa powder
- ✓ 2 tbsp pure date sugar

Directions:

- ❖ Set a silicone egg tray aside. Puree the cranberries, date syrup, and vanilla in a blender until smooth.
- ❖ Add the cashew cream and plant butter to a medium pot. Heat over medium heat until the mixture is well combined. Turn the heat off. Mix in the cranberry mixture and divide the mixture into the muffin holes. Refrigerate for 40 minutes or until firm. Remove the tray and pop out the truffles.
- ❖ Meanwhile, mix the cocoa powder and date sugar on a plate. Roll the truffles in the mixture until well dusted and serve

80) COCONUT PEACH TART

Preparation Time: 10 minutes		Servings: 8

Ingredients:

- ✓ ½ cup rolled oats
- ✓ 1 cup cashews
- ✓ 1 cup soft pitted dates
- ✓ 1 cup canned coconut milk
- ✓ 2 large peaches, chopped
- ✓ ½ cup shredded coconut

Directions:

- ❖ In a food processor, pulse the oats, cashews, and dates until a dough-like mixture forms. Press down into a greased baking pan.
- ❖ Pulse the coconut milk, ½ cup water, peaches, and shredded coconut in the food processor until smooth. Pour this mixture over the crust and spread evenly. Freeze for 30 minutes. Soften 15 minutes before serving. Top with whipped coconut cream and shredded coconut

81) TROPICAL MANGO MUFFINS WITH CHOCOLATE CHIPS

Preparation Time: 40 minutes		Servings: 12

Ingredients:

- ✓ Ingredients for 12 servings
- ✓ 2 medium mangoes, chopped
- ✓ 1 cup non-dairy milk
- ✓ 2 tbsp almond butter
- ✓ 1 tsp apple cider vinegar
- ✓ 1 tsp pure vanilla extract
- ✓ 1 ¼ cups whole-wheat flour
- ✓ ½ cup rolled oats
- ✓ ¼ cup coconut sugar
- ✓ 1 tsp baking powder
- ✓ ½ tsp baking soda
- ✓ ½ cup unsweetened cocoa powder
- ✓ ¼ cup sesame seeds
- ✓ A pinch of salt
- ✓ ¼ cup dark chocolate chips

Directions:

- ❖ Preheat oven to 360 F.
- ❖ In a food processor, put the mangoes, milk, almond butter, vinegar, and vanilla. Blend until smooth.
- ❖ In a bowl, combine the flour, oats, sugar, baking powder, baking soda, cocoa powder, sesame seeds, salt, and chocolate chips. Pour into the mango mixture and mix. Scoop into greased muffin cups and bake for 20-25 minutes. Let cool completely before removing from the cups

82) EASY MAPLE RICE PUDDING

Preparation Time: 30 minutes		Servings: 4

Ingredients:

- ✓ 1 cup short-grain brown rice
- ✓ 1 ¾ cups non-dairy milk
- ✓ 4 tbsp pure maple syrup
- ✓ 1 tsp vanilla extract
- ✓ A pinch of salt
- ✓ ¼ cup dates, pitted and chopped

Directions:

- ❖ In a pot over medium heat, place the rice, milk, 1 ½ cups water, maple, vanilla, and salt. Bring to a boil, then reduce the heat. Cook for 20 minutes, stirring occasionally. Mix in dates and cook for another 5 minutes. Serve chilled in cups

83) DELICIOUS VANILLA COOKIES WITH POPPY SEEDS

Preparation Time: 15 minutes		Servings: 3

Ingredients:

- ✓ ¾ cup plant butter, softened
- ✓ ½ cup pure date sugar
- ✓ 1 tsp pure vanilla extract
- ✓ 2 tbsp pure maple syrup
- ✓ 2 cups whole-grain flour
- ✓ ¾ cup poppy seeds, lightly toasted

Directions:

- ❖ Beat the butter and sugar in a bowl until creamy and fluffy. Add in vanilla, and maple syrup, blend. Stir in flour and poppy seeds. Wrap the dough in a cylinder and cover it with plastic foil. Let chill in the fridge.
- ❖ Preheat oven to 330 F. Cut the dough into thin circles and arrange on a baking sheet. Bake for 12 minutes, until light brown. Let completely cool before serving

84) BEST KIWI AND PEANUT BARS

Preparation Time: 5 minutes		Servings: 9

Ingredients:

- ✓ 2 kiwis, mashed
- ✓ 1 tbsp maple syrup
- ✓ ½ tsp vanilla extract
- ✓ 2 cups old-fashioned rolled oats
- ✓ ½ tsp salt
- ✓ ¼ cup chopped peanuts

Directions:

- ❖ Preheat oven to 360 F.
- ❖ In a bowl, add kiwi, maple syrup, and vanilla and stir. Mix in oats, salt, and peanuts. Pour into a greased baking dish and bake for 25-30 minutes, until crisp. Let completely cool and slice into bars to serve

85) SPECIAL TROPICAL CHEESECAKE

Preparation Time: 20 minutes + cooling time | | **Servings:** 4

Ingredients:

- ✓ 2/3 cup toasted rolled oats
- ✓ ¼ cup plant butter, melted
- ✓ 3 tbsp pure date sugar
- ✓ 6 oz cashew cream cheese
- ✓ ¼ cup coconut milk
- ✓ 1 lemon, zested and juiced
- ✓ ¼ cup just-boiled water
- ✓ 3 tsp agar agar powder
- ✓ 1 ripe mango, chopped

Directions:

- ❖ Process the oats, butter, and date sugar in a blender until smooth.
- ❖ Pour the mixture into a greased 9-inch springform pan and press the mixture onto the bottom of the pan. Refrigerate for 30 minutes until firm while you make the filling.
- ❖ In a large bowl, using an electric mixer, whisk the cashew cream cheese until smooth. Beat in the coconut milk, lemon zest, and lemon juice. Mix the boiled water and agar agar powder until dissolved and whisk this mixture into the creamy mix. Fold in the mango.
- ❖ Remove the cake pan from the fridge and pour in the mango mixture. Shake the pan to ensure a smooth layering on top. Refrigerate further for at least 3 hours. Remove the cheesecake from the fridge, release the cake pan, slice, and serve

86) ENGLISH RAISIN OATMEAL BISCUITS

Preparation Time: 20 minutes | | **Servings:** 8

Ingredients:

- ✓ ½ cup plant butter
- ✓ 1 cup date sugar
- ✓ ¼ cup pineapple juice
- ✓ 1 cup whole-grain flour
- ✓ 1 tsp baking powder
- ✓ ½ tsp salt
- ✓ 1 tsp pure vanilla extract
- ✓ 1 cup old-fashioned oats
- ✓ ½ cup vegan chocolate chips
- ✓ ½ cup raisins

Directions:

- ❖ Preheat oven to 370 F. Beat the butter and sugar in a bowl until creamy and fluffy. Pour in the juice and blend. Mix in flour, baking powder, salt, and vanilla. Stir in oats, chocolate chips, and raisins. Spread the dough on a baking sheet and bake for 15 minutes. Let completely cool on a rack

87) EXOTIC COCONUT AND CHOCOLATE BROWNIES

Preparation Time: 40 minutes | | **Servings:** 4

Ingredients:

- ✓ 1 cup whole-grain flour
- ✓ ½ cup unsweetened cocoa powder
- ✓ 1 tsp baking powder
- ✓ ½ tsp salt
- ✓ 1 cup pure date sugar
- ✓ ½ cup canola oil
- ✓ ¾ cup almond milk
- ✓ 1 tsp pure vanilla extract
- ✓ 1 tsp coconut extract
- ✓ ½ cup vegan chocolate chips
- ✓ ½ cup sweetened shredded coconut

Directions:

- ❖ Preheat oven to 360 F. In a bowl, combine the flour, cocoa, baking powder, and salt.
- ❖ In another bowl, whisk the date sugar and oil until creamy. Add in almond milk, vanilla, and coconut extracts. Mix until smooth. Pour into the flour mixture and stir to combine. Fold in the coconut and chocolate chips. Pour the batter into a greased baking pan and bake for 35-40 minutes. Let cool before serving

88) RICH EVERYDAY ENERGY BARS

Preparation Time: 35 minutes | | **Servings:** 16

Ingredients:

- ✓ 1 cup vegan butter
- ✓ 1 cup brown sugar
- ✓ 2 tbsp agave syrup
- ✓ 2 cups old-fashioned oats
- ✓ 1/2 cup almonds, slivered
- ✓ 1/2 cup walnuts, chopped
- ✓ 1/2 cup dried currants
- ✓ 1/2 cup pepitas

Directions:

- ❖ Begin by preheating your oven to 320 degrees F. Line a baking pan with parchment paper or Silpat mat.
- ❖ Thoroughly combine all the ingredients until everything is well incorporated.
- ❖ Spread the mixture onto the prepared baking pan using a wide spatula.
- ❖ Bake for about 33 minutes or until golden brown. Cut into bars using a sharp knife and enjoy

89) HEALTHY RAW COCONUT ICE CREAM

Preparation Time: 10 minutes + chilling time | | **Servings:** 2

Ingredients:

- ✓ 4 over-ripe bananas, frozen
- ✓ 4 tbsp coconut milk
- ✓ 6 fresh dates, pitted
- ✓ 1/4 tsp pure coconut extract
- ✓ 1/2 tsp pure vanilla extract
- ✓ 1/2 cup coconut flakes

Directions:

- ❖ Place all the ingredients in the bowl of your food processor or high-speed blender.
- ❖ Blitz the ingredients until creamy or until your desired consistency is achieved.
- ❖ Serve immediately or store in your freezer.
- ❖ Enjoy

90) DELICIOUS CHOCOLATE HAZELNUT FUDGE

Preparation Time: 1 hour 10 minutes | | **Servings:** 20

Ingredients:

- ✓ 1 cup cashew butter
- ✓ 1 cup fresh dates, pitted
- ✓ 1/4 cup cocoa powder
- ✓ 1/4 tsp ground cloves
- ✓ 1 tsp matcha powder
- ✓ 1 tsp vanilla extract
- ✓ 1/2 cup hazelnuts, coarsely chopped

Directions:

- ❖ Process all ingredients in your blender until uniform and smooth.
- ❖ Scrape the batter into a parchment-lined baking sheet. Place it in your freezer for at least 1 hour to set.
- ❖ Cut into squares and serve. Enjoy

91) ENGLISH OATMEAL SQUARES WITH CRANBERRIES

Preparation Time: 25 minutes | | **Servings:** 20

Ingredients:

- ✓ 1 ½ cups rolled oats
- ✓ 1/2 cup brown sugar
- ✓ 1 tsp baking soda
- ✓ A pinch of coarse salt
- ✓ A pinch of grated nutmeg
- ✓ 1/2 tsp cinnamon
- ✓ 2/3 cup peanut butter
- ✓ 1 medium banana, mashed
- ✓ 1/3 cup oat milk
- ✓ 1 tsp vanilla extract
- ✓ 1/2 cup dried cranberries

Directions:

- ❖ Begin by preheating your oven to 350 degrees F.
- ❖ In a mixing bowl, thoroughly combine the dry ingredients. In another bowl, combine the wet ingredients.
- ❖ Then, stir the wet mixture into the dry ingredients; mix to combine well.
- ❖ Spread the batter mixture in a parchment-lined baking pan. Bake in the preheated oven for about 20 minutes.
- ❖ Let it cool on a wire rack. Cut into squares and enjoy

92) TRADITIONAL BREAD PUDDING WITH SULTANAS

Preparation Time: 2 hours | | **Servings:** 4

Ingredients:

- ✓ 10 ounces day-old bread, cut into cubes
- ✓ 2 cups coconut milk
- ✓ 1/2 cup coconut sugar
- ✓ 1 tsp vanilla extract
- ✓ 1/2 tsp ground cloves
- ✓ 1/2 tsp ground cinnamon
- ✓ 1/2 cup Sultanas

Directions:

- ❖ Place the bread cubes in a lightly oiled baking dish.
- ❖ Now, blend the milk, sugar, vanilla, ground cloves and cinnamon until creamy and smooth.
- ❖ Spoon the mixture all over the bread cubes, pressing them with a wide spatula to soak well; fold in Sultanas and set aside for about 1 hour.
- ❖ Bake in the preheated oven at 350 degrees F for about 1 hour or until the top of your pudding is golden brown.
- ❖ Enjoy

93) ORIGINAL DECADENT HAZELNUT HALVAH

Preparation Time: 10 minutes | | **Servings:** 16

Ingredients:

- ✓ 1/2 cup tahini
- ✓ 1/2 cup almond butter
- ✓ 1/4 cup coconut oil, melted
- ✓ 4 tbsp agave nectar
- ✓ 1/2 tsp pure almond extract
- ✓ 1/2 tsp pure vanilla extract
- ✓ 1/8 tsp salt
- ✓ 1/8 tsp freshly grated nutmeg
- ✓ 1/2 cup hazelnuts, chopped

Directions:

- ❖ Line a square baking pan with parchment paper.
- ❖ Mix the ingredients, except for the hazelnuts, until everything is well incorporated.
- ❖ Scrape the batter into the parchment-lined pan. Press the hazelnuts into the batter.
- ❖ Place in your freezer until ready to serve. Enjoy

94) TASTY ORANGE MINI CHEESECAKES

Preparation Time: 10 minutes + chilling time | | **Servings:** 12

Ingredients:

- ✓ Crust:
- ✓ 1 cup raw almonds
- ✓ 1 cup fresh dates, pitted
- ✓ Topping:
- ✓ 1/2 cup raw sunflower seeds, soaked overnight and drained
- ✓ 1 cup raw cashew nuts, soaked overnight and drained
- ✓ 1 orange, freshly squeezed
- ✓ 1/4 cup coconut oil, softened
- ✓ 1/2 cup dates, pitted
- ✓ Garnish:
- ✓ 2 tbsp caramel topping

Directions:

- ❖ In your food processor, blend the crust ingredients until the mixture comes together; press the crust into a lightly greased muffin tin.
- ❖ Then, blend the topping ingredients until creamy and smooth. Spoon the topping mixture onto the crust, creating a flat surface with a spatula.
- ❖ Place these mini cheesecakes in your freezer for about 3 hours. Garnish with caramel topping. Enjoy

95) EASY BERRY COMPOTE WITH RED WINE

Preparation Time: 15 minutes | | **Servings:** 4

Ingredients:

- ✓ 4 cups mixed berries, fresh or frozen
- ✓ 1 cup sweet red wine
- ✓ 1 cup agave syrup
- ✓ 1/2 tsp star anise
- ✓ 1 cinnamon stick
- ✓ 3-4 cloves
- ✓ A pinch of grated nutmeg
- ✓ A pinch of sea salt

Directions:

- ❖ Add all ingredients to a saucepan. Cover with water by 1 inch. Bring to a boil and immediately reduce the heat to a simmer.
- ❖ Let it simmer for 9 to 11 minutes. Allow it to cool completely.
- ❖ Enjoy

---

96) TURKISH-STYLE IRMIK HELVASI

Preparation Time: 35 minutes | | **Servings:** 8

Ingredients:

- ✓ 1 cup semolina flour
- ✓ 1/2 cup coconut, shredded
- ✓ 1/2 tsp baking powder
- ✓ A pinch of salt
- ✓ 1 tsp pure vanilla extract
- ✓ 1 cup vegan butter
- ✓ 1 cup coconut milk
- ✓ 1/2 cup walnuts, ground

Directions:

- ❖ Thoroughly combine the flour, coconut, baking powder, salt and vanilla. Add in the butter and milk; mix to combine.
- ❖ Fold in the walnuts and let it rest for about 1 hour.
- ❖ Bake in the preheated oven at 350 degrees F for approximately 30 minutes or until a tester inserted in the center of the cake comes out dry and clean.
- ❖ Transfer to a wire rack to cool completely before slicing and serving. Enjoy

---

97) AUTHENTIC GREEK KOUFETO

Preparation Time: 15 minutes | | **Servings:** 8

Ingredients:

- ✓ 1 pound pumpkin
- ✓ 8 ounces brown sugar
- ✓ 1 vanilla bean
- ✓ 3-4 cloves
- ✓ 1 cinnamon stick
- ✓ 1 cup almonds, slivered and lightly toasted

Directions:

- ❖ Bring the pumpkin and brown sugar to a boil; add in the vanilla, cloves and cinnamon.
- ❖ Stir continuously to prevent from sticking.
- ❖ Cook until your Koufeto has thickened; fold in the almonds; let it cool completely. Enjoy

98) WINTER TANGY FRUIT SALAD WITH LEMON DRESSING

Preparation Time: 15 minutes		Servings: 4

Ingredients:

- ✓ Salad:
- ✓ 1/2 pound mixed berries
- ✓ 1/2 pound apples, cored and diced
- ✓ 8 ounces red grapes
- ✓ 2 kiwis, peeled and diced
- ✓ 2 large oranges, peeled and sliced
- ✓ 2 bananas, sliced
- ✓ Lemon Dressing:
- ✓ 2 tbsp fresh lemon juice
- ✓ 1 tsp fresh ginger, peeled and minced
- ✓ 4 tbsp agave syrup

Directions:

- ❖ Mix all the ingredients for the salad until well combined.
- ❖ Then, in a small mixing bowl, whisk all the lemon dressing ingredients.
- ❖ Dress your salad and serve well chilled. Enjoy

99) EUROPEAN GERMAN-STYLE APPLE CRUMBLE

Preparation Time: 50 minutes		Servings: 8

Ingredients:

- ✓ 4 apples, cored, peeled and sliced
- ✓ 1/2 cup brown sugar
- ✓ 1 cup all-purpose flour
- ✓ 1/2 cup coconut flour
- ✓ 2 tbsp flaxseed meal
- ✓ 1 tsp baking powder
- ✓ 1/2 tsp baking soda
- ✓ A pinch of sea salt
- ✓ A pinch of freshly grated nutmeg
- ✓ 1/2 tsp ground cinnamon
- ✓ 1/2 tsp ground anise
- ✓ 1/2 tsp pure vanilla extract
- ✓ 1/2 tsp pure coconut extract
- ✓ 1 cup coconut milk
- ✓ 1/2 cup coconut oil, softened

Directions:

- ❖ Arrange the apples on the bottom of a lightly oiled baking pan. Sprinkle brown sugar over them.
- ❖ In a mixing bowl, thoroughly combine the flour, flaxseed meal, baking powder, baking soda, salt, nutmeg, cinnamon, anise, vanilla and coconut extract.
- ❖ Add in the coconut milk and softened oil and mix until everything is well incorporated. Spread the topping mixture over the fruit layer.
- ❖ Bake the apple crumble at 350 degrees F for about 45 minutes or until golden brown. Enjoy

100) DELICIOUS VANILLA CINNAMON PUDDING

Preparation Time: 25 minutes		Servings: 4

Ingredients:

- ✓ 1 cup basmati rice, rinsed
- ✓ 1 cup water
- ✓ 3 cups almond milk
- ✓ 12 dates, pitted
- ✓ 1 tsp vanilla paste
- ✓ 1 tsp ground cinnamon

Directions:

- ❖ Add the rice, water and 1 ½ cups of milk to a saucepan. Cover the saucepan and bring the mixture to a boil.
- ❖ Turn the heat to low; let it simmer for another 10 minutes until all the liquid is absorbed.
- ❖ Then, add in the remaining ingredients and stir to combine. Let it simmer for 10 minutes more or until the pudding has thickened. Enjoy

101) FRESH MINT CHOCOLATE CAKE

Preparation Time: 45 minutes | | **Servings:** 16

Ingredients:

- ✓ 1/2 cup vegan butter
- ✓ 1/2 cup brown sugar
- ✓ 2 chia eggs
- ✓ 3/4 cup all-purpose flour
- ✓ 1 tsp baking powder
- ✓ A pinch of salt
- ✓ A pinch of ground cloves
- ✓ 1 tsp ground cinnamon
- ✓ 1 tsp pure vanilla extract
- ✓ 1/3 cup coconut flakes
- ✓ 1 cup vegan chocolate chunks
- ✓ A few drops peppermint essential oil

Directions:

- ❖ In a mixing bowl, beat the vegan butter and sugar until fluffy.
- ❖ Add in the chia eggs, flour, baking powder, salt, cloves, cinnamon and vanilla. Beat to combine well.
- ❖ Add in the coconut and mix again.
- ❖ Scrape the mixture into a lightly greased baking pan; bake at 350 degrees F for 35 to 40 minutes.
- ❖ Melt the chocolate in your microwave and add in the peppermint essential oil; stir to combine well.
- ❖ Afterwards, spread the chocolate ganache evenly over the surface of the cake. Enjoy

102) ORIGINAL OLD-FASHIONED COOKIES

Preparation Time: 45 minutes | | **Servings:** 12

Ingredients:

- ✓ 1 cup all-purpose flour
- ✓ 1 tsp baking powder
- ✓ A pinch of salt
- ✓ A pinch of grated nutmeg
- ✓ 1/2 tsp ground cinnamon
- ✓ 1/4 tsp ground cardamom
- ✓ 1/2 cup peanut butter
- ✓ 2 tbsp coconut oil, room temperature
- ✓ 2 tbsp almond milk
- ✓ 1/2 cup brown sugar
- ✓ 1 tsp vanilla extract
- ✓ 1 cup vegan chocolate chips

Directions:

- ❖ In a mixing bowl, combine the flour, baking powder and spices.
- ❖ In another bowl, combine the peanut butter, coconut oil, almond milk, sugar and vanilla. Stir the wet mixture into the dry ingredients and stir until well combined.
- ❖ Fold in the chocolate chips. Place the batter in your refrigerator for about 30 minutes. Shape the batter into small cookies and arrange them on a parchment-lined cookie pan.
- ❖ Bake in the preheated oven at 350 degrees F for approximately 11 minutes. Transfer them to a wire rack to cool slightly before serving. Enjoy

103) DELICIOUS COCONUT CREAM PIE

Preparation Time: 15 minutes + chilling time | | **Servings:** 12

Ingredients:

- ✓ Crust:
- ✓ 2 cups walnuts
- ✓ 10 fresh dates, pitted
- ✓ 2 tbsp coconut oil at room temperature
- ✓ 1/4 tsp groin cardamom
- ✓ 1/2 tsp ground cinnamon
- ✓ 1 tsp vanilla extract
- ✓ Filling:
- ✓ 2 medium over-ripe bananas
- ✓ 2 frozen bananas
- ✓ 1 cup full-fat coconut cream, well-chilled
- ✓ 1/3 cup agave syrup
- ✓ Garnish:
- ✓ 3 ounces vegan dark chocolate, shaved

Directions:

- ❖ In your food processor, blend the crust ingredients until the mixture comes together; press the crust into a lightly oiled baking pan.
- ❖ Then, blend the filling layer. Spoon the filling onto the crust, creating a flat surface with a spatula.
- ❖ Transfer the cake to your freezer for about 3 hours. Store in your freezer.
- ❖ Garnish with chocolate curls just before serving. Enjoy

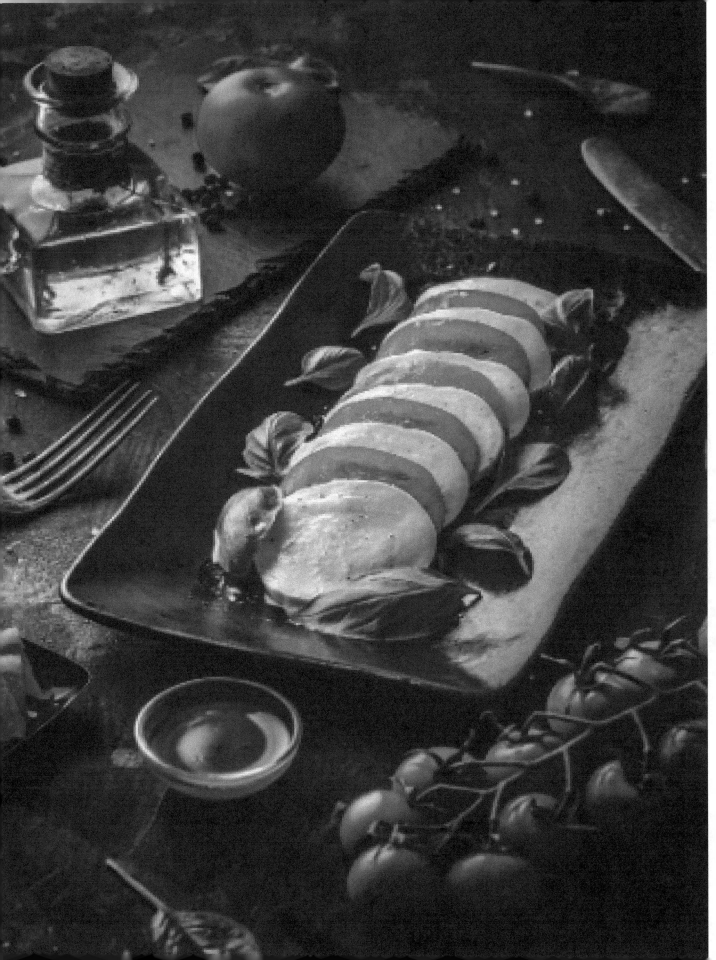

1) 3 series X 15 **CRUNCHES** (Stop for 30" from each series)

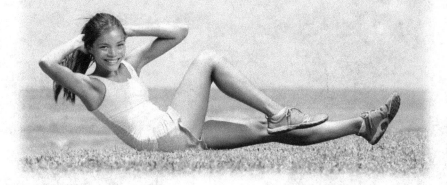

2) 2 series X 30 **BICYCLE CRUNCHES** (Stop for 30" from each series)

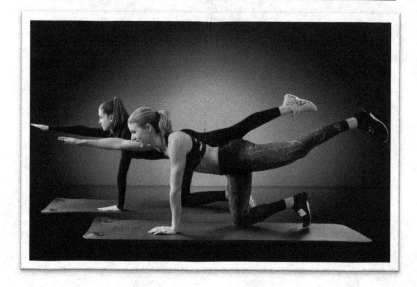

3) 3 series X 20

ALTERNATING LEG AND ARM EXTENSION QUADRUPED

(Stop for 10" from each series)

4) 3 series X 20 **CROSS BODY** (Stop for 10" from each series)

In plank position up your left leg and cross it with the right side. Repeat with the other side.

5) 2 series X 15" **PLANK SIDEWALK** (Stop for 10" from each series)

In plank position, move yourself: the first step with left leg on the left; then the second step with the right leg on the left. Make 3 complete steps and return at the beginning place, making steps one by one on the right.

6) 2 series X 10 **PRESS-UPS** (Stop for 30" from each series)

7) 2 series X 30" **SIDE LEG CIRCLES** (Stop for 10" from each series)

Lie down on the left side. Up your right leg and move it in a circle for 30". Turn yourself and repeat with the other leg.

8) 3 series X 20 **SQUATS** (Stop for 30" from each series)

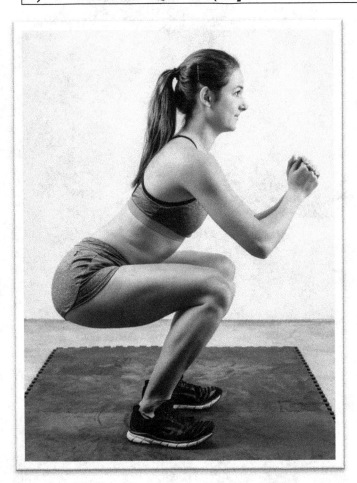

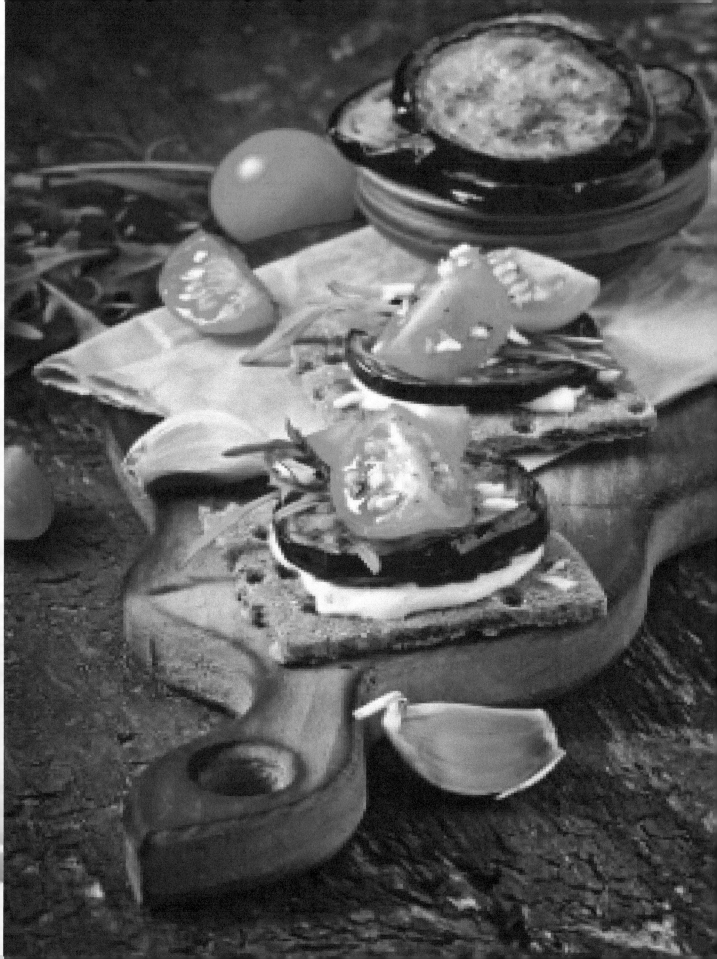

Bibliography

FROM THE SAME AUTHOR

THE VEGETARIAN DIET *Cookbook* - 100+ Easy-to-Follow Recipes for Beginners! TASTE Yourself with the Most Vibrant Plant-Based Cuisine Meals!

THE VEGETARIAN DIET FOR ATHLETES *Cookbook* - The Best Recipes for Athletic Performance and Muscle Growth! More Than 100 High-Protein Plant-Based Meals to Maintain a Perfect Body!

THE VEGETARIAN DIET FOR BEGINNERS *Cookbook* - 100+ Super Easy Recipes to Start a Healthier Lifestyle! The Best Recipes You Need to Jump into the Tastiest Plant-Based World!

THE VEGETARIAN DIET FOR MEN *Cookbook* - The Best 100 Recipes to Stay FIT! Sculpt Your Abs Before Summer with the Healthiest Plant-Based Meals!

THE VEGETARIAN DIET FOR WOMEN *Cookbook* - The Best 100 recipes to stay TONE and HEALTHY! Reboot your Metabolism before Summer with the Tastiest and Lightest Plant-Based Meals!

THE VEGETARIAN DIET FOR KIDS *Cookbook* - The Best 100 recipes for children, tested BY Kids FOR Kids! Jump into the Plant-Based World to Stay Healthy HAVING FUN!

THE VEGETARIAN DIET FOR WOMEN OVER 50 *Cookbook* - The Best Plant-Based Recipes to Restart Your Metabolism! Maintain the Right Hormonal Balance and Lose Weight with More Than 100 Light and Healthy Recipes!

THE VEGETARIAN DIET FOT MEN OVER 50 *Cookbook* - The Best Recipes to Restart Your Metabolism! Stay Healthy with More than 100 Easy and Mouthwatering Recipes!

Conclusion

Thanks for reading "Vegetarian Diet for Women *Cookbook*"!

Follow the right habits it is essential to have a healthy Lifestyle, and the Vegetarian diet is the best solution!

I hope you liked this Cookbook!

I wish you to achieve all your goals!

Jocelyn Grant

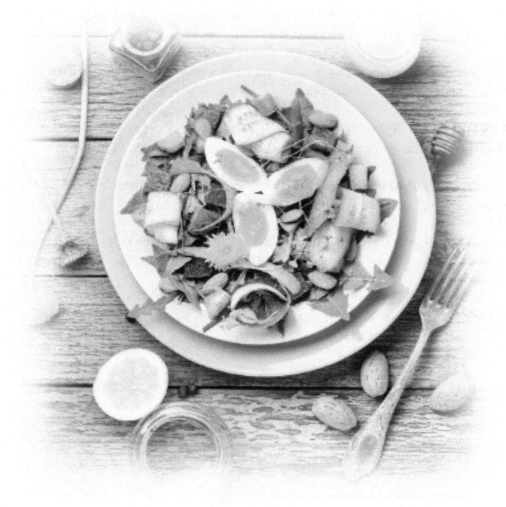